SpringerBriefs in Statistics

T0238851

For further volumes:
http://www.springer.com/series/8921

George A. F. Seber · Mohammad M. Salehi

Adaptive Sampling Designs

Inference for Sparse
and Clustered Populations

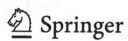
Springer

George A. F. Seber
Department of Statistics
University of Auckland
Auckland
New Zealand

Mohammad M. Salehi
Department of Mathematics,
 Statistics and Physics
Qatar University
Doha
Qatar

ISSN 2191-544X
ISBN 978-3-642-33656-0
DOI 10.1007/978-3-642-33657-7
Springer Heidelberg New York Dordrecht London

ISSN 2191-5458 (electronic)
ISBN 978-3-642-33657-7 (eBook)

Library of Congress Control Number: 2012949064

Printed on acid-free paper

Springer is part of Springer Science+Business Media (www.springer.com)

Preface

Animal populations are always challenging to sample especially if the animals are rare or if they occur in clusters that are widely dispersed, such as schools of fish. Ordinary sampling methods tend to fail because animals generally get missed. In 1988 and the early 1990s, Steven Thompson published several important papers that introduced a new way of sampling called adaptive cluster sampling. This method used the information coming in during the sampling to change the way further sampling was to be carried out. Since those early papers there has an upsurge of research on the topic covering a wide range of underlying populations in addition to animal populations. In this monograph we consider not only this work but also other "adaptive methods" such as sequential and inverse sampling and methods of allocating further sample observations that come under the umbrella of so-called "adaptive allocation". Our main focus is on the sampling design and design-based estimation and not model-base estimation where the underlying observations are assume to follow some statistical distribution as in a "super-population" approach.

Since the subject is fairly extensive and can be complex at times, one aim in writing this monograph is to get across the basic ideas and the supporting mathematics for those unfamiliar with the subject matter. Our second aim is to give a review of the literature for those wishing to carry out research on the topic.

The reader is assumed to have some basic ideas about sampling from a finite population such as simple random sampling and stratification. Chapter 1 deals briefly with some popular types of sampling designs and the role of adaptive methods. An important technique called adaptive cluster sampling is introduced in Chap. 2 and various methods of estimation along with confidence intervals are given. Chapter 3 summarizes some of the foundational theory behind adaptive sampling including the Rao–Blackwell theorem for improving the efficiency of estimation. The role of primary and secondary units, including stratified and two-stage adaptive sampling, is considered in Chap. 4. The last two Chaps. 5 and 6 focus on a range of adaptive allocation methods including inverse sampling and two-stage procedures.

Auckland, New Zealand, October 2012   George A. F. Seber
Doha, Qatar, October 2012   Mohammad M. Salehi

Contents

Chapter 1
Basic Ideas

Abstract In this chapter we consider the problem of estimating such quantities as the number of objects, the total biomass, or total ground cover in a finite population from a sample. Various traditional methods of sampling such as sampling with or without replacement, inverse sampling, and unequal probability sampling are often inadequate when the population is rare but clustered. We briefly introduce the idea of adaptive sampling that includes a variety of so-called adaptive methods. For example, adaptive cluster sampling allows us to sample the rest of a cluster when one is located. We can also have adaptive allocation in stratified sampling where the initial observations in the strata determine the allocation of future observations.

Keywords Adaptive sampling · Adaptive cluster sampling · Adaptive cluster double sampling · Unequal probability sampling · Adaptive allocation · Stratified sampling

1.1 The Estimation Problem

In its simplest form, the main problem we are interested in is estimating the total number, mean number, or density of certain objects (e.g., animals) in a population of area A. A general method is to divide up the population into N plots or *units* and then sample some of the units. The units can have a variety of shapes including squares and circles. If y_i $(i = 1, 2, \ldots, N)$ is the number of objects in the ith unit, then we are interested in estimating the total $\tau = \sum_{i=1}^{N} y_i$, the mean per unit $\mu = \tau/N$, the density $D = \tau/A$, or some other function of the population y-values. Here y_i can be continuous (e.g., biomass, pollution level) or discrete (e.g., number of plants or animals), and this includes an indicator variable which takes the value of 1 if a certain characteristic is present in the unit or 0 if it is absent.

G. A. F. Seber and M. M. Salehi, *Adaptive Sampling Designs*, SpringerBriefs in Statistics, DOI: 10.1007/978-3-642-33657-7_1, © The Author(s) 2013

1.1.1 Examples

The types of additional problems that one can meet are seen in the following examples.

Example 1. Suppose y_i is the total area of plot i covered by a certain species of plant so that D now becomes the proportion of the population covered by the plant. If we are interested in k species of plants and y_{ij} is the measurement for the jth species, then y_i now becomes a k-dimensional vector $\mathbf{y}_i = (y_{i1}, y_{i2} \ldots, y_{ik})'$. This can lead to comparing the abundances of various species.

Example 2. Sometimes a population area has certain well defined regions or strata that may affect the distribution of the objects. For example, heavy ground cover that can act as camouflage, or difficult terrain, may affect the distribution of a small animal. In this case the strata generally need to be considered separately by having plots in each stratum and then the results can be combined in some way.

Example 3. A powerful technique that can be used for designing experiments and determining how many plots should be sampled is the method of two-stage sampling. Here the population is divided up into larger plots called primary units and then each primary unit is divided into smaller plots or secondary units. The sampling method is to first choose a sample of primary units (stage 1) and then in each of those chosen units choose a sample of secondary units (stage 2). The number of primary units selected largely helps us to determine how accurate we want our final estimate to be. Also the units in a primary unit need not be contiguous (together).

Example 4. Different shapes can be used for plots. For example, strip transects are frequently used as the sampling unit in wildlife studies (e.g., aerial and ship surveys of animals and marine mammals). Each strip can be regarded as a "primary" unit that is then divided into smaller plots to simplify the counting. Other shapes can be used.

Example 5. Suppose we have a population of animals, but not all animals are seen on a unit. In this case we can introduce the notion of the probability of detection, and the theory can be modified accordingly to allow for incomplete detectability.

1.2 Sampling Designs

We now consider some of the more common methods of choosing a sample of n_1 units from the population of N units. These are referred to as sampling designs and do not require any assumptions about the population, for example whether it is randomly dispersed or not. In the latter case of random dispersion, the y_i observations can be modeled by a statistical distribution. This approach will be discussed briefly in Sect. 1.5 below.

1.2.1 Traditional Designs

The most common design is choosing a unit at random without replacement after each selection, usually referred to as simple random sampling. A second method used in some situations is sampling with replacement, where a particular unit can be chosen more than once. A third design uses a form of systematic sampling with a random start. A fourth design uses unequal probability sampling, as in sampling a tree with probability proportional to its basal area. A fifth design is inverse sampling where units are sampled without replacement until the sum of the y-values reaches or exceeds a prescribed value. A sixth design called sequential sampling typically involves choosing a first sample, then, on the basis of the information obtained, a second sample is drawn as well. A number of variations of this method are available. We now provide some theory for simple random sampling, unequal probability sampling, and stratified sampling for later use.

1.2.2 Simple Random Sampling

Suppose $\bar{y}$ is the mean of the y values obtained from simple random sample of n units. Then, from standard theory (e.g., Cochran 1977; Thompson 2002) $E[\bar{y}] = \mu$ and

$$\text{var}[\bar{y}] = \frac{1}{n} \cdot \frac{1}{N-1} \sum_{i=1}^{N} (y_i - \mu)^2 \left(1 - \frac{n}{N}\right), \tag{1.1}$$

with unbiased estimate

$$\widehat{\text{var}}[\bar{y}] = \frac{1}{n} \cdot \frac{1}{n-1} \sum_{i=1}^{n_1} (y_i - \bar{y})^2 \left(1 - \frac{n}{N}\right). \tag{1.2}$$

Note that we have followed a standard misuse of notation where we have treated the sample of values as $y_1, y_2, \ldots, y_n$ instead of $y_{i_1}, y_{i_2}, \ldots, y_{i_n}$.

1.2.3 Unequal Probability Sampling

Suppose that the N population units are labeled $i = 1, 2, \ldots, N$, and we have a sample of fixed size n selected without replacement using any sampling design for which the selection probability of unit i is p_i in the first draw ($i = 1, 2, \ldots, N$). Let $s_R = \{i_1, i_2, \ldots, i_n\}$ denote the unordered sequence of distinct labels in the sample (we use s_R instead of s because of a later extension in Chap. 5), and let d_R denote the observed unordered set of distinct pairs (i, y_i) in the sample so that

$d_R = \{(i, y_i) : i \in s_R\}$. Murthy (1957) obtained the following estimator of μ, namely

$$\widehat{\mu}_M = \frac{1}{N} \sum_{i=1}^n y_i \frac{P(s_R \mid i)}{P(s_R)}, \tag{1.3}$$

where $P(s_R \mid i)$ denotes the conditional probability of getting sample s_R, given the ith unit was selected first. From Murthy (1957),

$$\mathrm{var}[\widehat{\mu}_M] = \frac{1}{N^2} \sum_{i=1}^N \sum_{j<i}^N \left(1 - \sum_{s_R \ni i,j} \frac{P(s_R \mid i) P(s_R \mid j)}{P(s_R)}\right) \left(\frac{y_i}{p_i} - \frac{y_j}{p_j}\right)^2 p_i p_j, \tag{1.4}$$

with unbiased estimator

$$\widehat{\mathrm{var}}[\widehat{\mu}_M] = \frac{1}{N^2} \sum_{i=1}^n \sum_{j<i}^n \left(\frac{P(s_R \mid i, j)}{P(s_R)} - \frac{P(s_R \mid i) P(s_R \mid j)}{[P(s_R)]^2}\right) \left(\frac{y_i}{p_i} - \frac{y_j}{p_j}\right)^2 p_i p_j, \tag{1.5}$$

where $P(s_R \mid i, j)$ denotes the probability of getting the sample s_R given that the units i and j were selected (in either order) in the first two draws. Using the theory of Chap. 3 we shall show in Sect. 5.2 that Murthy's estimator can be applied to quite general sampling designs.

Under the umbrella of unequal probability sampling there are two other estimators that can be used in certain situations, namely the Horvitz-Thompson and Hansen-Hurwitz estimators. Modifications of these estimators are considered in the next chapter for adaptive cluster sampling.

1.2.4 Stratified Sampling

Suppose the population area is divided into H strata with N_h units in stratum h ($h = 1, 2, \ldots, H$) and $N = \sum_{h=1}^H N_h$, the total number of population units. Let y_{ih} be the y-value for unit i in stratum h, and let μ_h be the mean of the y-values for stratum h. We assume that any sampling is carried out independently in each stratum. If $\widehat{\mu}_h$ is an unbiased estimate of μ_h based on the sample in stratum h, and $\widehat{\mathrm{var}}[\widehat{\mu}_h]$ is an unbiased estimate of $\mathrm{var}[\widehat{\mu}_h]$, then we have the following unbiased estimate of μ for the whole population and an unbiased estimate of its variance, namely

$$\widehat{\mu} = \sum_{h=1}^H \frac{N_h}{N} \widehat{\mu}_h \quad \text{and} \quad \widehat{\mathrm{var}}[\widehat{\mu}] = \sum_{h=1}^H \frac{N_h^2}{N^2} \widehat{\mathrm{var}}[\widehat{\mu}_h]. \tag{1.6}$$

If $\widehat{\mu}_h = \overline{y}_h$ is the sample mean of a simple random sample of n_h observations in stratum h, then from (1.1),

$$\text{var}[\widehat{\mu}] = \frac{1}{N^2} \sum_{h=1}^{H} N_h(N_h - n_h)\frac{\sigma_h^2}{n_h}, \tag{1.7}$$

where[1]

$$\sigma_h^2 = \frac{1}{N_h - 1} \sum_{i=1}^{N_h}(y_{hi} - \mu_h)^2$$

is the population variance of the y-values for stratum h. An unbiased estimate of $\text{var}[\widehat{\mu}]$ is given by replacing each σ_h^2 by its unbiased estimate

$$s_h^2 = \frac{1}{n_h - 1} \sum_{i=1}^{n_h}(y_{hi} - \overline{y}_h)^2.$$

If we are able to take $n = \sum_{h=1}^{H} n_h$ observations altogether, an important question is how do we allocate the n_h to minimise $\text{var}[\widehat{\mu}]$. The answer is given by the so-called Neyman allocation $n_h \propto N_h\sigma_h$, or

$$n_h = n\frac{N_h\sigma_h}{\sum_{r=1}^{H} N_r\sigma_r}. \tag{1.8}$$

The above theory for stratified sampling can be found in any standard sampling book (e.g., Cochran 1977; Thompson et al. 1992).

1.2.5 Some Problems

Problems can arise with the above methods for some populations, especially if the individuals are rare or elusive. General methods for handling such problem populations are discussed by various authors in Thompson (2004). In particular, if a population is sparse but clustered, for example a fish population forming large widely scattered schools with few fish in between, then using simple random sampling may lead to a lot of empty plots with schools largely missed. With inverse sampling an unreasonably large number of units might need to be sampled. To get round this problem of missed clusters, one approach is to use a method called adaptive sampling, the main topic of this book.

---

[1] We use the traditional divisor $N_h - 1$ instead of N_h as it simplifies expressions.

1.3 Adaptive Sampling

One aspect of adaptive sampling can be described very simply as follows. We go fishing in a lake using a boat and, assuming complete ignorance about the population, we select a location at random and fish. If we don't catch anything we select another location at random and try again. If we do catch something, we fish in a specific neighborhood of that location and keep expanding the neighborhood until we catch no more fish. We then move on to a second selected location. This process continues until we have, for example, fished at a fixed number of initial locations or until our total catch has exceeded a certain number of fish. In brief, adaptive sampling refers to adapting the sampling pattern to what turns up at each stage of the sampling process. Such a method can be applied to each of the five examples in Sect. 1.1.1. Another method of locating more individuals is to simply increase the size of a sample plot by a fixed factor when a certain criterion is satisfied by the sample plot (Yang et al. 2011).

1.3.1 Adaptive Cluster Sampling

The most popular of the adaptive methods is adaptive cluster sampling developed by Thompson (1988, 1990, 2002). A review of the topic from 1990 to 2003 is given by Turk and Borkowski (2005). We now describe this design mathematically using the notation of Thompson and Seber (1996). It consists of (1) defining a neighborhood where further sampling might be carried out, (2) defining a condition for choosing when to sample the neighborhood, and (3) choosing a method for selecting the initial locations.

A neighborhood of a unit can be defined in a number of ways and have a variety of patterns. For example, a simple neighborhood of a unit i could consist of adjacent units (e.g., plots) with a common boundary which, together with unit i, form a "cross." Although the units in a neighborhood do not have to be next to each other, they must have a "symmetry" property, so that if unit j is in the neighborhood of unit i, then unit i is in the neighborhood of unit j.

The next step is specify a condition C such as $y_i > c$ that determines when we sample the neighborhood of the ith plot; typically $c = 0$ if y_i is a count. If C for the ith unit is satisfied, we sample all the units in its neighborhood and if the rule is satisfied for any of those units we sample their neighborhoods as well, and so on, thus leading to a cluster of units. This cluster has the property that all the units on its "boundary" (called "edge units") do not satisfy C. Because of a dual role played by the edge units, the underlying theory is based on the concept of a network for unit i, which is the cluster minus its edge units. We denote it by A_i. It should be noted that if the initial unit selected is any one of the units in the cluster except an edge unit, then all the units in the cluster end up being sampled. Thus some of the A_i are duplicated. The choice of c for the condition C is critical. If it is too low it can lead to a "feast" of plots, while if it is too high it can lead to a "famine."

If the unit selected is an edge unit, C is not satisfied and there is no augmentation so that we have a cluster of one unit. The same is true for any other selected unit that doesn't satisfy C. This means that all clusters of size one are also networks of size one. Thus any cluster consisting of more than one unit can be split into a network and further networks of size 1 (one for each edge unit). In contrast to having clusters that may overlap on their edge units, the distinct networks are disjoint and form a partition of the N units.

If a unit is chosen at random, the probability of selecting the cluster it belongs to will depend on the size of the cluster. For this reason adaptive cluster sampling can be described as unequal probability cluster sampling—a form of biased sampling.

The final step is to decide on n_1 the size of the initial sample. Each time we select an initial unit we add to it adaptively so that the final number of units selected, n say, will be a random variable. The usual methods for selecting an initial sample are sampling either with or without replacement, and these two designs are considered in the next chapter. We shall see later, however, that all of the sampling designs mentioned in Sect. 1.2 have been used in various situations.

1.3.2 Adaptive Cluster Double Sampling

Félix-Medina and Thompson (2004) proposed an extension of the above method that they called adaptive cluster double sampling. It requires the availability of an inexpensive and easy-to-measure auxiliary variable (e.g., a so-called "rapid-assessment"variable) that is used to select a first-phase adaptive cluster sample. The network structure of this first-phase sample is used to select the subsequent subsamples, which are selected using conventional designs. For example, we can choose a first-phase random sample of networks from those initially selected (or use all those networks) and then take a conventional second-phase subsample from each of the selected networks. One variation is to omit the second phase altogether. We only record the y-values of the units in the final-phase subsample. This scheme has the following advantages: (1) the number of y-measurements can controlled, (2) the final sample is near places of interest, (3) the second-phase sampling can be started before the first-phase sampling is completed, and (4) the auxiliary variable can be used to construct a regression-type estimator. Muttlak and Khan (2002) consider a similar scheme in which large clusters are sampled, but small clusters are fully included.

1.3.3 Stratified Sampling

Sometimes we have prior information about how a population is dispersed so that we can divide up the population area into distinct areas or *strata*. We can then carry out adaptive cluster sampling in each stratum and either truncate the adaptive process at each stratum boundary or allow the clusters to overlap boundaries. These two scenarios are discussed in Sect. 4.5.

1.3.4 Adaptive Allocation

In stratified sampling, one of the difficulties is to determine the optimal way of allocating observations to each stratum since we find from Eq. (1.8) that this involves knowing the stratum population variances. These can be estimated using past survey information or else using a pilot survey so that the sampling is effectively done in two phases. Variance estimates from the initial stages (phase 1) can be used to allocate further samples in a sequential fashion (phase 2). For example, we can choose a stratum at each stage of phase 2 to give the greatest reduction in the overall estimated variance. The phase-2 allocation is, in this sense, adaptive. A simple two-phase design would be to take a simple random selection of units in each stratum for the first phase and then return to those strata with, say, the largest y-values and sample more units.

The main problem with the above methods is that they require two "passes" over the population area. Here the first pass provides the phase-1 sample, and this determines the phase-2 sampling effort in the second pass. An alternative method is to use one pass in a sequential fashion. The strata are sampled one at a time in a particular order with the level of sampling in a particular stratum depending on what happens in the preceding stratum. Some theory for adaptive allocation methods is given in Chap. 6.

1.4 Related Methods

We observe that inverse and sequential sampling can be regarded as adaptive methods of sampling, but with the sample size rather than the method of selecting the units being adaptive. We note that the network (multiplicity) sampling introduced by Sirken (1970) and others (see Kalton and Anderson 1986, for references) is different from adaptive sampling, though they both use the idea of a network. Snowball sampling, a form of adaptive sampling, has also been suggested as a potential method in the detection and study of rare or hidden human populations (Kalton and Anderson 1986). For further comments the reader is referred to Sect. 2.5.

1.5 Model-Based Methods

Our focus in this monograph is on design-based estimation where any distribution theory used is based solely on the randomness of the sampling method, that is on the sampling design used. Sometimes it is not possible to use an appropriate form of random sampling in selecting sample units. There are two alternative ways of dealing with this problem. If one is simply interested in numbers of objects so that y_i is the number of objects in unit i, then one can make assumptions about the spatial distribution of the objects. The simplest assumption is that the objects are randomly distributed so that we find that the joint distribution of the y_i is multinomial and the sum of the sampled y-values is binomial. If the individuals tend to be clustered, one can use a distribution like the negative binomial distribution (Seber 2002, pp. 450–451). If the y_i are measurements, then a model-based approach assumes that $\mathbf{y} = (y_1, y_2, \dots, y_N)'$ is the observed value of a random vector with a specified distribution such as, for example, the multivariate normal or lognormal distribution. This underlying stochastic model is sometimes refereed to as a "super population" and the theoretical foundations of this approach are set out in Thompson and Seber (1996, Chap. 3). In comparing the design- and model-based approaches Rapley and Welsh (2008) make the following comment:

> At a pragmatic level, in very simple, general terms, the design-based approach trades off efficiency for wide applicability while the model-based approach which is usually more efficient when the assumed model holds, trades off wide applicability for increased efficiency.

In the case of adaptive sampling, Rapley and Welsh combine both the design- and model-based methods using a Bayesian approach. For an example using Poisson modeling see Thompson et al. (1992) and Thompson and Seber (1996, pp. 196–199).

1.6 Optimal Designs

It is well-known that, with a design-based approach, there is no sampling strategy that is uniformly optimal over all possible (unknown) y-values (Godambe 1955; Godambe and Joshi 1965). However, under a population stochastic model, an optimal design strategy often does exist and in general it is an adaptive one (Thompson and Seber 1996, pp. 236–237). An adaptive sample is essentially a multi-phase design where the "phase" of a survey is defined as a point at which a selection of units may be made based on what has already been observed. This occurs every time an initial sample unit is chosen. The simplest such scheme is a two-phase design where one chooses an initial sample of n_1 units (non-adaptively) and the result of this is used to determine a further sample of n_2 units, a method we have called adaptive allocation in Chap. 6. Thompson and Seber (1996, pp. 237–240) showed that under a stochastic population model, an optimal two-phase procedure does at least as good as using an optimal conventional design with sample size $n_1 + n_2$ in terms of mean-square error. This theory is applied to the case where $\mathbf{y}_i$ is an observation from a known multivariate lognormal distribution by Chao and Thompson (2001). Chao (2003) also provides a strategy for the two-phase model.

References

Chao, C-T. 2003. "Markov Chain Monte Carlo on Optimal Adaptive Sampling Selections." *Environmental and Ecological Statistics* 10(1):129–151.

Chao, C-T., and S.K. Thompson. 2001."Optimal Adaptive Selection of Sampling Sites". *Environmetrics*12:517–538.

Cochran W.G. 1977. *Sampling Techniques*, 3rd edit. New York: Wiley.

Félix-Medina M.H., and S.K. Thompson. 2004. "Adaptive Cluster Double Sampling." *Biometrika* 91:877–891.

Godambe V.P. 1955. "A Unified Theory of Sampling from Finite Populations." *Journal of the Royal Statistical Society, Series B* 17:269–278.

Godambe V.P., and V.M. Joshi. 1965. "Admissibility and Bayes Estimation." *Annals of Mathematical Statistics* 36:1701–1722.

Kalton G., and D.W. Anderson. 1986. "Sampling Rare Populations." *Journal of the Royal Statistical Society, Series A* 147:65–82.

Muttlak H.A., and A. Khan. 2002. "Adjusted Two-stage Adaptive Cluster Sampling." *Environmental and Ecological Statistics* 9:111–120.

Murthy, M.N. 1957. "Ordered and Unordered Estimators in Sampling Without Replacement." *Sankhyā* 18:379–390.

Rapley, V.E., and A.H. Welsh. 2008. "Model-based Inferences from Adaptive Cluster Sampling." *Bayesian, Analysis* 3(4):717–736.

Seber, G. A. F. 1982. *The Estimation of Animal Abundance and Related Parameters*, 2nd edit.London: Griffin. Reprinted by Blackburn Press, Caldwell, New Jersey, U.S.A. (2002).

Sirken, M.G. 1970. "Household Surveys with Multiplicity." *Journal of the American Statistical Association* 63:257–266.

Thompson, S.K. 1988. "Adaptive Sampling." In *Proceedings of the Section on Survey Research Methods of the American Statistical Association*, 784–786.

Thompson, S.K. 1990. "Adaptive Cluster Sampling". *Journal of the American Statistical Association* 85:1050–1059.

Thompson, S.K. 2002. *Sampling*, 2nd edit. New York.

Thompson, S.K., F.L. Ramsey, and G.A.F. Seber. 1992. "An Adaptive Procedure for Sampling Animal Populations." *Biometrics* 48:1196–1199.

Thompson, S.K., and G.A.F. Seber. 1996. *Adaptive Sampling*. New York: Wiley.

Thompson, W.L. (Ed.) 2004. *Sampling Rare or Elusive Species: Concepts, Designs, and Techniques for Estimating Population Parameters*. Washington, DC: Island Press.

Turk, P., and J.J. Borkowski. 2005. "A Review of Adaptive Cluster Sampling: 1990–2003." *Environmental and Ecological Statistics* 12:55–94.

Yang, H., C. Kleinn, L. Fehrmann, S. Tang, and S. Magnussen. 2011. A New Design for Sampling with Adaptive Sample Plots. *Environmental and Ecological Statistics* 18:223–237.

Chapter 2
Adaptive Cluster Sampling

Abstract One of the main methods of adaptive sampling is adaptive cluster sampling. As it involves unequal probability of sampling, standard Horvitz-Thompson and Hansen-Hurwitz estimators can be modified to provide unbiased estimates of finite population parameters along with unbiased variance estimators. These estimators are compared with each other and with conventional estimators. Confidence intervals are discussed, including bootstrap and empirical likelihood methods, and a biased estimator that we call Hájek's estimator is described because of its link with this topic. The chapter closes with some theory about selecting networks without replacement.

Keywords Indicator variables · Horvitz-Thompson estimator · Hansen-Hurwitz estimator · Bootstrap · Hájek's estimator · Empirical likelihood confidence interval · Networks selected without replacement

2.1 Unbiased Estimation

2.1.1 Notation

In addition to estimating the population mean $\mu = \sum_{1=1}^{N} y_i / N$ of the population y-values, we shall also be interested in estimating the population variance defined as $\sigma^2 = \sum_{i=1}^{N} (y_i - \mu)^2 / (N - 1)$. We consider taking a simple random sample of size n_1 and adding adaptively to give a final sample of size n, which will be a random variable. As adaptive cluster sampling (ACS) is essentially about sampling clusters, we shall consider two methods, sampling clusters with or without replacement. As the size of a cluster determines its probability of selection, we find, not surprisingly, that the standard Horvitz-Thompson (Horvitz and Thompson 1952) and Hansen-Hurwitz (Hansen and Hurwitz 1943) estimators for unequal probability sampling can be modified to provide unbiased estimators. We now consider these below. But first we introduce some theory of indicator functions.

G. A. F. Seber and M. M. Salehi, *Adaptive Sampling Designs*, SpringerBriefs in Statistics, 11
DOI: 10.1007/978-3-642-33657-7_2, © The Author(s) 2013

2.1.2 Indicator Variables

Let I_j ($j = 1, 2, \ldots, r$) be an indicator variable that takes the value 1 with probability π_j and 0 with probability $1 - \pi_j$. Then $I_j I_k$ is also an indicator variable taking the value of 1 with probability π_{jk}, where

$$
\begin{aligned}
\pi_{jk} &= P([J_j = 1] \cap [J_k = 1]) \\
&= P(I_j = 1) + P(I_k = 1) - P([I_j = 1] \cup [I_k = 1]) \\
&= P(I_j = 1) + P(I_k = 1) - (1 - P([I_i \neq 1] \cap [I_j \neq 1])).
\end{aligned} \tag{2.1}
$$

As we shall see below, we are often interested in finding the mean and variance of an expression like

$$
Z = \sum_{j=1}^{r} z_j I_j, \tag{2.2}
$$

where the z_j are constants. To do this we first note that I_j is a binomial random variable based on a single binomial trial so that $E[I_j] = \pi_j$ and $\mathrm{var}[I_j] = \pi_j(1-\pi_j)$. Also

$$
\mathrm{cov}[I_j, I_k] = E[I_j I_k] - E[I_j]E[I_k] = \pi_{jk} - \pi_j \pi_k. \tag{2.3}
$$

Hence

$$
E[Z] = \sum_{j=1}^{r} z_j E[I_j] = \sum_{j=1}^{r} z_j \pi_j, \tag{2.4}
$$

and

$$
\begin{aligned}
\mathrm{var}[Z] &= \sum_{j=1}^{r} \sum_{k=1}^{r} z_j z_k \mathrm{cov}[I_j, I_k] \\
&= \sum_{j=1}^{r} z_j^2 \mathrm{var}[I_j] + \sum_{j=1}^{r} \sum_{k \neq j} z_j z_k \mathrm{cov}[I_j, I_k] \\
&= \sum_{j=1}^{r} z_i^2 \pi_j(1 - \pi_j) + \sum_{j=1}^{r} \sum_{k \neq j} z_j z_k (\pi_{jk} - \pi_j \pi_k) \\
&= \sum_{j=1}^{r} \sum_{k=1}^{r} z_j z_k (\pi_{jk} - \pi_j \pi_k),
\end{aligned} \tag{2.5}
$$

with the convention that $\pi_{jj} = \pi_j$. Since $\mathbf{I}_j^2 = \mathbf{I}_j$, an unbiased estimate of $\mathrm{var}[Z]$ is given by

$$\widehat{\text{var}}[Z] = \sum_{j=1}^{r} z_j^2 (1 - \pi_j) I_j + \sum_{j=1}^{r} \sum_{k \neq j} \frac{(\pi_{jk} - \pi_j \pi_k)}{\pi_{jk}} I_j I_k$$

$$= \sum_{j=1}^{r} \sum_{k=1}^{r} z_j z_k I_j I_k \left(\frac{\pi_{jk} - \pi_j \pi_k}{\pi_{jk}} \right). \tag{2.6}$$

2.1.3 Modified Horvitz-Thompson (HT) Estimator

We begin by taking an initial random sample of units without replacement. Since clusters can overlap on their edge units, we avoid this problem by using networks. We recall from Sect. 1.3.1 that A_i is the network of units (the cluster minus its edge units) associated with unit i, and it has m_i units, say. Since every item in a network will lead to the same network being selected, we effectively have some networks selected with replacement. In order to use the Horvitz-Thompson estimator we need to know the probability of selection of each unit in the final sample. Unfortunately these probabilities are only known for units in networks selected by the initial sample, and not for the edge units attached to these networks, as an edge unit may belong to another unselected cluster. Therefore, in what follows, we ignore all edge units that are not in the initial sample and use only network information when it comes to computing the final estimators.

Suppose there are K distinct networks in the population forming a partition of the population, and let x_k ($k = 1, 2, \ldots, K$) be the number of units in the kth network. Note that all the m_i will be the same and equal to x_k for every unit i in the kth network. If α_k is the probability of selecting the kth network, then it is the probability of selecting any unit in that network so that $\alpha_i = \alpha_k$ for every unit i in network k. Thompson (1990) proposed the following estimator, which is of the form of Z in the previous section, namely

$$\widehat{\mu}_{HT} = \frac{1}{N} \sum_{i=1}^{K} \frac{y_k^* J_k}{\alpha_k}$$

$$= \frac{1}{N} \sum_{k=1}^{\kappa} \frac{y_k^*}{\alpha_k}, \tag{2.7}$$

where y_k^* is the sum of the y-values for the kth network, κ is the number of distinct networks in the sample, and J_k is an indicator variable taking the value of 1 (with probability α_k) if the initial sample intersects the kth network, and 0 otherwise. If p_k is the probability that the kth network is not selected, then

$$\alpha_k = 1 - p_k = 1 - \left[\binom{N - x_k}{n_1} \middle/ \binom{N}{n_1} \right]. \tag{2.8}$$

Hence

$$E[\widehat{\mu}_{HT}] = \frac{1}{N} \sum_{k=1}^{K} y_k^* = \frac{1}{N} \sum_{i=1}^{N} y_i = \mu,$$

showing that $\widehat{\mu}_{HT}$ is an unbiased estimate. To find its variance, we require the probabilities p_{jk} that the jth and kth networks are not intersected and α_{jk} the probability that both are intersected. Then

$$p_{jk} = P([J_j \neq 1] \cap [J_k \neq 1])$$
$$= \binom{N - x_j - x_k}{n_1} \bigg/ \binom{N}{n_1},$$

and, from (2.1),

$$\alpha_{jk} = \alpha_j + \alpha_k - (1 - p_{jk})$$
$$= 1 - \left[\binom{N - x_j}{n_1} + \binom{N - x_k}{n_1} - \binom{N - x_j - x_k}{n_1} \right] \bigg/ \binom{N}{n_1}. \quad (2.9)$$

We now substitute π for α, z_j for y_j^*/α_j in the previous section and obtain

$$\text{var}[\widehat{\mu}_{HT}] = \frac{1}{N^2} \left[\sum_{j=1}^{K} \sum_{k=1}^{K} y_j^* y_k^* \left(\frac{\alpha_{jk} - \alpha_j \alpha_k}{\alpha_j \alpha_k} \right) \right], \quad (2.10)$$

with an unbiased estimate

$$\widehat{\text{var}}[\widehat{\mu}_{HT}] = \frac{1}{N^2} \left[\sum_{j=1}^{K} \sum_{k=1}^{K} y_j^* y_k^* \left(\frac{\alpha_{jk} - \alpha_j \alpha_k}{\alpha_{jk} \alpha_j \alpha_k} \right) J_j J_k \right]$$
$$= \frac{1}{N^2} \left[\sum_{j=1}^{K} \sum_{k=1}^{K} \frac{y_j^* y_k^*}{\alpha_{jk}} \left(\frac{\alpha_{jk}}{\alpha_j \alpha_k} - 1 \right) \right], \quad (2.11)$$

where α_{jj} is interpreted as α_j.

The estimator $\widehat{\mu}_{HT}$ can be expressed in the form (Thompson and Seber 1996, pp. 95–97)

$$\widehat{\mu}_{HT} = \frac{1}{N} \sum_{i=1}^{N} y_i \frac{J_i'}{E[J_i']}, \quad (2.12)$$

where $J_i' = 1$ if the initial sample intersects A_i and 0 otherwise. This shows that the estimator is also unbiased if sampling is with replacement. We then still have (2.10) and (2.11) but with

$$\alpha_k = 1 - \left(1 - \frac{x_k}{N}\right)^{n_1},$$

and

$$\alpha_{jk} = 1 - \left\{\left(1 - \frac{x_j}{N}\right)^{n_1} + \left(1 - \frac{x_k}{N}\right)^{n_1} - \left(1 - \frac{x_j + x_k}{N}\right)^{n_1}\right\}.$$

We observe that all the above selection probabilities of the networks depend on n_1. This means that we can't use a pilot survey to try and determine the size of n_1 to achieve a certain accuracy. We come back to this problem when we consider two-stage sampling in Chap. 4.

2.1.4 Modified Hansen-Hurwitz (HT) Estimator

Another estimator proposed by Thompson (1990) is a generalization of the Hansen-Hurwitz (HH) estimator, namely

$$\widehat{\mu}_{HH} = \frac{1}{N} \sum_{i=1}^{N} y_i \frac{f_i}{E[f_i]}, \tag{2.13}$$

where f_i is the number of units in the initial sample that fall in (intersect) the network A_i. This estimate is clearly unbiased. Once again ignoring the edge units of clusters in the estimation process, f_i is the number of times that the ith unit in the final sample occurs in the estimator. We note that $f_i = 0$ if no units in the initial sample intersect A_i. The above equation refers to a weighted sum of all the y-values in the final sample *including repeats*, where the weight $1/E[f_i]$ is the same for every unit in A_i. Since the f_i units are selected from the m_i units in A_i, f_i has a hypergeometric distribution with parameters (N, m_i, n_1) so that $E[f_i] = n_1 m_i / N$. Combining these two ideas,

$$\widehat{\mu}_{HH} = \frac{1}{n_1} \sum_{i=1}^{N} \frac{y_i f_i}{m_i}$$

$$= \frac{1}{n_1} \sum_{i=1}^{n_1} \frac{1}{m_i} \sum_{j \in A_i} y_j$$

$$= \frac{1}{n_1} \sum_{i=1}^{n_1} w_i$$

$$= \overline{w}, \quad \text{say}, \tag{2.14}$$

where w_i is the mean of the m_i observations in A_i (Thompson 1990). It follows from Eqs. (1.1) and (1.2) that

$$\text{var}[\widehat{\mu}_{HH}] = \frac{N - n_1}{Nn_1(N - 1)} \sum_{i=1}^{N}(w_i - \mu)^2, \tag{2.15}$$

with unbiased estimate

$$\widehat{\text{var}}[\widehat{\mu}_{HH}] = \frac{N - n_1}{Nn_1(n_1 - 1)} \sum_{i=1}^{n_1}(w_i - \widehat{\mu}_{HH})^2. \tag{2.16}$$

We now give another form for $\widehat{\mu}_{HH}$. Since w_i ($= \bar{v}_k$, say) is the same for each unit in the kth network, we have

$$\widehat{\mu}_{HH} = \frac{1}{n_1} \sum_{k=1}^{\kappa} b_k \bar{v}_k,$$

where b_k is the number of times the kth network appears in $\widehat{\mu}_{HH}$, and κ is the number of distinct networks intercepted by the initial sample. Since $b_k = 0$ for those networks not intersected and has a hypergeometric distribution with parameters (N, x_k, n_1) otherwise, $E[b_k] = n_1 x_k / N$ and

$$\begin{aligned} \widehat{\mu}_{HH} &= \frac{1}{n_1} \sum_{k=1}^{K} b_k \bar{v}_k \\ &= \frac{1}{n_1} \sum_{k=1}^{K} \frac{b_k y_k^*}{x_k} \\ &= \frac{1}{N} \sum_{k=1}^{K} y_k^* \frac{b_k}{E[b_k]}, \end{aligned} \tag{2.17}$$

where y_k^* is the sum of the y-values in the kth network. We see then that $\widehat{\mu}_{HH}$ can be expressed in terms of units or networks. Examples showing the calculation of the HT and HH estimators (defined as $\widehat{\mu}$ and $\widetilde{\mu}$ respectively) are given by Thompson and Seber (1996, pp. 113–117).[1]

From (2.13) we see that $\widehat{\mu}_{HH}$ is still unbiased when sampling is with replacement. As $f_i \sim \text{Bin}(n_1, m_i/n)$, we still have $\text{Ex}[f_i] = n_1 m_i / N$. This means that (2.14) is still the same and $\widehat{\mu}_{HH}$ is still a sample mean, but for sampling with replacement. We can define a random variable W that takes the value w_i with probability $1/N$, so that

$$\sigma_W^2 = \text{var}[W] = \sum_{i=1}^{N}(w_i - \mu)^2 P(W = w_i) = \frac{1}{N} \sum_{i=1}^{N}(w_i - \mu)^2.$$

---

[1] See also http://www.cee.vt.edu/ewr/environmental/teach/smprimer/adaptive/adaptv.html.

Hence

$$\text{var}[\widehat{\mu}_{HH}] = \text{var}[\overline{w}] = \frac{\sigma_W^2}{n_1}$$

with unbiased estimator

$$\widehat{\text{var}}[\widehat{\mu}_{HH}] = \frac{1}{n_1(n_1 - 1)} \sum_{i=1}^{n_1} (w_i - \widehat{\mu}_{HH})^2.$$

Both of the above HT and HH estimators were proposed by Thompson (1990).

2.1.5 Comparison of the HT and HH Estimators

These two estimators have been compared by Salehi (2003) and further comments about their corresponding confidence intervals are made in the Sect. 2.3 below. Both variances are unchanged by within-network variation because they involve the sum of the y-values over networks. However, as noted by Salehi, the within-network variation does affect the variance of the sample mean from a simple random sample (SRS) so that the relative efficiency of these adaptive estimators to SRS will increase as the within-network variance increases. In comparing the efficiencies of the two estimators, Salehi concludes that the HT estimator is preferred to the HH estimator from both theoretical considerations and from numerical examples provided by various authors. However the HH estimator and its unbiased variance estimator are easier to compute.

2.1.6 Efficiency Gains Over Conventional Methods

A number of writers have focused on the efficiency of estimators under ACS designs and indicate that they may be more efficient than conventional designs. The efficiency strongly depends on the spatial distribution of the population, and the efficiency gain is not guaranteed (e.g., Smith et al. 2004; Smith et al. 2003). As might be expected, an ACS design can significantly increase the likelihood of observing rare elements. The two factors that interact to determine the efficiency of ACS are the within network variance relative to the population variance and the final sample fraction relative to initial sample fraction (Thompson 1990; Smith et al. 1995). Adaptive cluster sampling, as with conventional cluster sampling, is efficient when the within network (or within cluster) variance is close to the population variance, which occurs when the population is clustered. Simultaneously, ACS is efficient when the final sample size is close to the initial sample size, which occurs when the population is rare. However, the two aims can be at odds with each other because small differences between initial and final sample size usually mean small within-network variance. Brown (2003) concludes that a compromise is needed so that "networks that are small enough to ensure the final sample size is not excessively large compared with the initial sample size but large enough to ensure the within-network variance is a reasonable fraction of the population variance."

ACS suffers from two problems: (1) its efficiency depends on the degree of rarity and clustering, which is unknown prior to sampling, and (2) the final sample size is unknown, which makes planning difficult. We can end up with too few observations so that the desired precision is not attained or there are too many observations (e.g., from a big cluster) that blow the survey budget! One way of getting of round this problem is to truncate the sampling at some point using a stopping rule, called restricted adaptive sampling (Brown and Manly 1998; Lo et al. 1997; Chao and Thompson 1999). This leads to biased estimators, which can be assessed using, for example, bootstrapping (Hanselman et al. 2003). The latter paper is an interesting study as it endeavors to look at a number of design problems such as choosing the criterion C. Brown and Manly (1998) estimated the biases using the bootstrap method and evaluated their method using simulation. They generated 27 populations with different degrees of patchiness. Bootstrapping was successful for removing the bias in only eight populations using the HT estimator and 17 populations using the HH estimator. Salehi and Seber (2002) presented unbiased estimators and their variance estimators for restricted adaptive cluster sampling and its without-replacement networks version. They found in their simulated example that the unbiased estimator had smaller mean-square errors than biased estimators for small sample sizes. However, the biased estimators had smaller mean-square errors when the final sample fractions are greater than 0.2.

Muttlak and Khan (2002) suggested an approach for populations in which some networks are large and others are small. After an initial simple random sample, subsamples are taken from the large networks, but the small networks are all included. Another recent method of trying to control the final sample size that has been applied to forestry is to simply enlarge a selected sample plot by a fixed factor when the criterion C is achieved on that plot (Yang et al. 2011).

2.1.7 Some Applications

Adaptive cluster sampling can be used for a wide diversity of populations. For example, Thompson and Seber (1996) described a number of applications to waterfowl, trees, contamination, household surveys for estimating rare characteristics (e.g., drug use, rare diseases), caterpillar infestations, and bark stripping by red deer. Some recent examples using ACS are: sediment load in rivers (Arabkhedri et al. 2010), larval sea lampreys (Sullivan et al. 2008), seaweed (Goldberg et al. 2006), herptofauna (Noon et al. 2006), trees (Roesch 1993; Magnussen et al. 2005; Talvitie et al. 2006; Acharya et al. 2000), plants (Acworth 1999; Philippi 2005; Ojiambo and Scherm 2010), pest density (Zhang et al. 2000), marsupials (Smith et al. 2004), hydroacoustic surveys (Conners and Schwager 2002), fish populations (Hanselman et al. 2003), fish eggs (Smith et al. 2004), sea urchins (Woodby 1998), fresh water mussels (Smith et al. 2011), thermal hotspots (Hung 2011), and robotics (Low et al. 2007).

2.1.8 Incomplete Detectability

Imperfect detectability is an issue when sampling rare species using adaptive cluster sampling. Detectability can influence the selection of adaptively sampled units because the condition to add more sampling units is typically based on a count of detected species. Thompson and Seber (1994) (see also Thompson and Seber 1996, Chap. 9) provided a solution to this problem by using estimated detection probabilities to correct estimates of population parameters. Smith et al. (2011) studied the effect of imperfect detectability on adaptive cluster sampling using a simulation study of freshwater mussels in the upper Mississippi River. The causes of imperfect detection in freshwater mussel surveys are varied. Some species are more cryptic (appear identical but are genetically quite distinct) or tend to be more endobenthic (living within the sediment on the seafloor) and are thus harder to detect than other more easily seen or epibenthic species (those living on the surface of the seafloor). Sampling was simulated using the computer program, SAMPLE, which can be down-loaded with documentation.[2] As expected it was found that, under perfect detection, estimates from conventional and adaptive designs were unbiased and adaptive sampling resulted in a higher probability of sampling occupied habitat than conventional sampling.

Imperfect detection caused biased estimates for both designs and degraded the relative performance of adaptive designs. Modified inclusion probabilities in adaptive cluster sampling are affected by imperfect detection. Nevertheless, bias in estimates was similar for conventional and adaptive designs. Adaptive sampling did result in encounter rates that exceeded those seen under conventional sampling. This finding arose because adaptive designs allocate sampling effort in the vicinity of clusters of individuals, such as mussel beds. However, this enhanced performance was degraded as detectability declined. Relative to conventional designs, adaptive sampling designs outperformed conventional designs on efficiency criterion only at the lowest density (0.2 mussels m^{-2}; rare species) when detection was imperfect.

2.2 Hájek's Estimator

We now introduce another estimator of the population mean μ that is mentioned below with regard to empirical likelihood confidence intervals. It uses the HT estimator but with an estimator of the population size N (whether it is known or not), and is given as follows:

$$\widehat{\mu}_{HJ} = \frac{1}{\widehat{N}} \sum_{i=1}^{K} \frac{y_k^* J_k}{\alpha_k} = \frac{1}{\widehat{N}} \sum_{k=1}^{\kappa} \frac{y_k^*}{\alpha_k}, \qquad (2.18)$$

---

[2] See http://www.lsc.usgs.gov/AEB/davids/acs/ for single stage, two stage, or stratified sampling.

where

$$\widehat{N} = \sum_{k=1}^{K} \frac{x_k}{\alpha_k}$$

is the HT estimator of N (i.e., we set $y_k = 1$) and x_k is the number of units in the kth network. Setting $z_k = y_k^* - x_k \mu$ and using Taylor linearization (sometimes refereed to as the delta-method), an approximate variance of $\widehat{\mu}_{HJ}$ is given by

$$\text{var}[\widehat{\mu}_{HJ}] \approx \frac{1}{N^2} \sum_{r=1}^{K} \sum_{s=1}^{K} (\alpha_{rs} - \alpha_r \alpha_s) \frac{z_r}{\alpha_r} \frac{z_s}{\alpha_s} \equiv V_{HJ}. \qquad (2.19)$$

An approximate estimator of V_{HJ} is

$$\widehat{V}_{HJ} = \frac{1}{N^2} \sum_{r=1}^{K} \sum_{s=1}^{K} \left(\frac{\alpha_{rs} - \alpha_r \alpha_s}{\alpha_{rs}} \right) \frac{\hat{z}_r}{\alpha_r} \frac{\hat{z}_s}{\alpha_s}, \qquad (2.20)$$

where $\hat{z}_k = y_k^* - x_k \widehat{\mu}_{HJ}$. The estimator $\widehat{\mu}_{HJ}$ is often attributed to Hájek (1971). For some self-weighting designs such as simple random sampling, $\widehat{\mu}_{HJ}$ and $\widehat{\mu}_{HT}$ are the same. The two estimators, however, are different for designs with unequal weights $1/\alpha_k$, and the unbiasedness of $\widehat{\mu}_{HJ}$ holds only approximately. In general, the Hájek estimator is less efficient than the HT estimator for a fixed sample size with α_k approximately proportional to the associated y-value. However, $\widehat{\mu}_{HJ}$ may be more efficient when the sample size is random (Särndal et al. 1992, p. 183).

2.3 Confidence Intervals

Di Consiglio and Scanu (2001) studied the asymptotic behaviors of $\widehat{\mu}_{HT}$ and $\widehat{\mu}_{HH}$ and proved that, under some complicated theoretical conditions, both estimators are asymptotically normally distributed. Using simulation they demonstrated that $\widehat{\mu}_{HT}$ can be approximately normal when the population is composed of a large number of segregated small clusters. On the other hand, $\widehat{\mu}_{HH}$ has the advantage of having the form of a sample mean (albeit for dependent observations) and requires less conditions for approximate normality, particularly when the cluster means are not widely different. When these estimators are based on small samples they often have highly skewed distributions. In such situations, confidence intervals based on traditional normal approximations can lead to unsatisfactory results, with poor coverage properties.

Félix-Medina (2003) showed that if the number of units in the initial sample as well as the number of units and networks in the population tend to infinity, but that the network sizes are bounded, then the HT and HH estimators are asymptotically normally distributed. He showed this for two cases: selecting the initial sample by simple random sampling without replacement and by unequal probability sampling with replacement.

2.3.1 Bootstrap Confidence Intervals

Christman and Pontius (2000) showed that bootstrap percentile methods are appropriate for constructing confidence intervals from the HH estimator. Perez and Pontius (2006) used the same methods as Christman and Pontius for constructing confidence intervals from the HH estimator. They showed that their bootstrap confidence intervals from the HT estimator are even worse than the normal approximation confidence intervals. Mohammadi (2011) proved that their bootstrap methods provide highly biased bootstrap estimates. He showed that the resampling techniques used by Perez and Pontius are inconsistent in the sense that they do not produce unbiased resample estimators and the bootstrap variances do not match the variance estimators. He proposed three bootstrap methods; a PPS Bootstrap With Replacement (BWR), simple BBW and the Gross's method (1980), which have those desired properties of unbiasedness and matching the variances. He developed bootstrap methods for $\widehat{\mu}_{HT}$ as well as $\widehat{\mu}_{HJ}$. His simulation study has shown that the bootstrap confidence intervals based on his proposed methods have better coverage intervals than those available from bootstrap methods and normal approximation.

2.3.2 Empirical Likelihood Confidence Intervals

Another non-parametric technique for constructing confidence intervals is the empirical likelihood method, using a non-parametric likelihood ratio function. The key idea behind this method is to restrict consideration to distributions with support on the observed data, making limited assumptions about the population distributions of the estimators without specifying a known parametric form. The method was first proposed by Hartley and Rao (1968) in the context of survey sampling and they called it the scale-load approach. Owen (1988) introduced this method under the name empirical likelihood as a device for constructing confidence intervals from independent observations.

Salehi et al. (2010) considered two pseudo empirical likelihood functions under the ACS design. One leads to $\widehat{\mu}_{HH}$ and the other to $\widehat{\mu}_{HJ}$. Based on these two empirical likelihood functions, they derived confidence intervals for the population mean. Using a simulation study, they showed that the confidence intervals obtained from the first empirical likelihood function perform as good as the bootstrap confidence intervals from $\widehat{\mu}_{HH}$, but the confidence intervals obtained from the second empirical likelihood function perform much better than the bootstrap confidence intervals from $\widehat{\mu}_{HT}$ used by Perez and Pontius (2006). A comparison between the empirical likelihood confidence intervals for $\widehat{\mu}_{HJ}$ and the bootstrap confidence intervals introduced by Mohammadi (2011) needs to be done.

2.4 Networks Selected Without Replacement

In the above adaptive cluster sampling (ACS) the number of distinct networks selected is random, as a network may be selected more than once. If the main sampling expense is the cost of traveling to the sites of the initial sample units, then we could control this cost better if we could fix the number of networks selected in advance. We now consider a sampling design in which, after each initial unit is selected, the corresponding network (which excludes its edge units) is "removed" from the population. The next initial unit is selected from what is left and we continue the process until we have selected n initial units thus giving n distinct networks without replacement.

Let x_k be the number of units in network k $(k = 1, 2, \ldots n)$, and define $y_k^* = \sum_{j=1}^{x_k} y_j$, the y-value of the network, and $w_k = y_k^*/x_k$, the mean of the y-values in network k. Then $\tau = \sum_{i=1}^{N} y_i = \sum_{k=1}^{k} y_k^*$ and $\mu = \tau/N$. We can use Murthy's estimator from Eq. (1.3) with the basic sampling unit now being the network (with y_i replaced by y_i^*). An unbiased estimate of μ is therefore

$$\widehat{\mu}_M = \frac{1}{N} \sum_{i=1}^{n} y_i^* \frac{P(s_R \mid i)}{P(s_R)},$$

where $P(s_R \mid i)$ denotes the conditional probability of getting sample s_R, given the ith network was selected first, s_R is the unordered sample of n networks, and $P(s_R \mid i)$ is the probability of choosing sample s_R given network i has been chosen as the first network. Now if p_i is the probability of getting network i in the first draw, we have $p_i = x_i/N$. Substituting in Eqs. (1.4) and (1.5) we get

$$\text{var}[\widehat{\mu}_M] = \frac{1}{N^2} \sum_{i=1}^{K} \sum_{j<i}^{K} x_i x_j \left(1 - \sum_{s_R \ni i, j} \frac{P(s_R \mid i) P(s_R \mid j)}{P(s_R)} \right) (w_i - w_j)^2,$$

with unbiased estimator

$$\widehat{\text{var}}[\widehat{\mu}_M] = \frac{1}{N^2} \sum_{i=1}^{n} \sum_{j<i}^{n} x_i x_j \left(\frac{P(s_R \mid i, j)}{P(s_R)} - \frac{P(s_R \mid i) P(s_R \mid j)}{[P(s_R)]^2} \right) (w_i - w_j)^2,$$

where $P(s_R \mid i, j)$ denotes the probability of getting the sample s_R given that the networks i and j were selected (in either order) in the first two draws. As the computation of $P(s_R)$ requires the consideration of $n!$ permutations, it is clear that in using

$\widehat{\mu}_M$ substantial computations are required when n is large. For further details see Salehi and Seber (1997). Estimators for the case of sampling without replacement of clusters rather than networks are given Dryver and Thompson (2006).

2.5 Further Extensions

We shall mention several extensions to the above theory. The first relates to the situation where the initial sample is no longer a simple random sample but is selected using unequal probability sampling, usually under the name of PPS sampling or probability proportional to size sampling. An important application of this is in forestry where trees are initially sampled with replacement and with probability proportional to the basal area of a tree. Adaptive sampling in forestry was proposed by Roesch (1993) who used circular neighborhoods. We can use the HT and HH estimators with different values for the network selection probabilities α_k and α_{rs} and for the expected frequencies $E[f_i]$. Details are given in Thompson and Seber (1996, pp. 100–108). For a general reference on tree sampling see Mandallaz (2008). Smith et al. (1995) also used a PPS method where the probability was proportional to the available habitat. The method can also be used in the selection of unequal sized primary units as for example in strip sampling (Pontius 1997).

A second application involves the use of order statistics. Here the observations from the initial sample of size n_1 taken without replacement are ordered according to their magnitude, namely $y_{(1)} < y_{(2)}, \ldots, < y_{(n_1)}$. We then decide to sample the neighborhoods of the units with the $(n_i - r)$ largest values, namely with y-values $y_{(r+1)}, y_{(r+2)}, \ldots, y_{(n_1)}$. Our criterion C for further adaptive sampling is $y_i \geq y_{(r+1)}$ which, in contrast to the above theory, now depends on the data. This sampling design, introduced by Thompson (1996), with simple examples, (see also Thompson and Seber 1996, pp. 164–175) is particularly useful for investigating pollution. Since the probability that the initial sample intersects the kth network depends on the other units in the sample, the HT estimator is no longer appropriate. However, the HH estimate is still unbiased and can be improved using the Rao-Blackwell theorem. Su and Quinn II (2003) used order statistics but with a stopping rule that led to biased estimators. The HT estimator was preferred as it was less sensitive to the stopping level.

One area of development relates to the problem of dealing with hidden human populations such as the Internet and other networked structures. These can be conceptualized mathematically as graphs and are hard to sample by conventional methods. The most effective sampling method is an adaptive one following links from one node to another, rather like a random walk. For some research related to this topic see Thompson (2006a,b). A related topic is link-tracing designs such as snowball sampling, random walk methods, and network sampling. These can be combined with adaptive sampling to sample hidden and hard-to-access human populations such as drug users, homeless persons, or undocumented worker populations (Thompson and Collins 2002). Model-based methods are particularly useful for such designs

(Thompson and Frank 2000; Félix-Medina and Thompson 2004). Bayesian models are discussed by Chow and Thompson (2003) and St. Clair and O'Connell (2011).

A natural extension of the above theory is the replacement of each observation y_i by a vector of observations $\mathbf{y}_i$. The above theory along with the Rao-Blackwell theorem can be readily applied to each of the jth elements of the $\mathbf{y}$ vectors independently. However, there are two main differences from the univariate case. First is the estimation of the covariances of the mean estimators and second is that the choice of the criterion C is not straightforward (Thompson 1993; Thompson and Seber 1996, Chap. 8; Dryver 2003). The effectiveness of the adaptive method depends on the relationships among the variables in the vectors and the formulation of the criterion C.

References

Acharya, B., A. Bhattarai, A. De Gier, and A. Stein. 2000. "Systematic Adaptive Cluster Sampling for the Assessment of Rare Tree Species in Nepal." *Forest Ecology and Management* 137:65–73.

Acworth, J. 1999. "Prunus Africana. Striving for Sustainable and Equitable Resource Management in Cameroon." *Medicinal Plant Conservation* 5:15–18.

Arabkhedri, M., F.S. Lai, I. Noor-Akma, and M.K. Mohamad-Roslan. 2010. "An Application of Adaptive Cluster Sampling for Estimating Total Suspended Sediment Load." *Hydrology Research* 41:63–73.

Brown, J.A. 2003. "Designing an Efficient Adaptive Cluster Sample." *Environmental and Ecological Statistics* 10:95–105.

Brown, J.A. and B.F.J. Manly. 1998. "Restricted Adaptive Cluster Sampling." *Environmental and Ecological Statistics* 5:49–63.

Chao, C-T., and S.K. Thompson. 1999. "Incomplete Adaptive Cluster Sampling Designs." In: *Proceedings of the Section on Survey Research Methods of the American Statistical Association*, 345–350.

Chow, M., and S.K. Thompson. 2003. "Estimation with Link-Tracing Sampling Designs: a Bayesian Approach." *Survey Methodology* 29:197–205.

Christman, M.C., and J.S. Pontius. 2000. "Bootstrap Confidence Intervals for Adaptive Cluster Sampling." *Biometrics* 56:503–510.

Conners, M.E., and S.J. Schwager. 2002. "The Use of Adaptive Cluster Sampling for Hydroacoustic Surveys." *ICES Journal of Marine Science* 59:1314–1325.

Di Consiglio, L.D., and M. Scanu. 2001. "Some Results on Asymptotics in Adaptive Cluster Sampling." *Statistics and Probability Letters* 52:189–197.

Dryver, A.L. 2003. "Performance of Adaptive Cluster Sampling Estimators in a Multivariate Setting." *Environmental and Ecological Statistics*. 10(1):107–113.

Dryver, A.L., and S.K. Thompson. 2006. " Adaptive Cluster Sampling without Replacement of Clusters." *Statistical Methodology* 4:35–43.

Félix-Medina, M.H. (2003). "Asymptotics in Adaptive Cluster Sampling." *Environmental and Ecological Statistics* 10:61–82.

Félix-Medina, M.H., and S.K. Thompson. 2004. "Combining Link-Tracing Sampling and Cluster Sampling to Estimate the Size of Hidden Populations." *Journal of Official Statistics* 20:19–38.

Goldberg, N.A., J.N. Heine, and J.A. Brown. 2006. "The Application of Adaptive Cluster Sampling for Rare Subtidal Macroalgae." *Marine Biology* 151:1343–1348.

Gross, S.T. 1980. "Median Estimation in Sample Surveys." In: *Proceedings of the Survey Research Methods Section*, 181–184. Alexandria, Virginia: American Statistical Association.

Hájek, J. 1971. "Comment on a paper by D. Basu." In: V.P. Godambe, and D.A. Sprott (eds.). *Foundations of Statistical Inference*, 236. Toronto: Holt, Rinehart and Winson.

Hanselman, D.H., T.J. Quinn II, C. Lunsford, J. Heifetz, and D. Clausen. 2003. "Applications in Adaptive Cluster Sampling of Gulf of Alaska Rockfish." *Fisheries Bulletin* 101:501–513.

Hansen, M.M., and W.N. Hurwitz. 1943. On the Theory of Sampling from Finite Populations." *Annals of Mathematical Statistics* 14:333–362.

Hartley H.O., and Rao J.N.K. 1968. "A New Estimation Theory for Sample Surveys." *Biometrika* 55:547–557.

Horvitz, D.G., D.J. Thompson. 1952. "A Generalization of Sampling Without Replacement from a Finite Universe." *Journal of the American Statistical Association* 47:663–685.

Hung, Y. 2011. "Adaptive Probability-Based Latin Hypercube Designs." *Journal of the American Statistical Association: Theory and Methods* 106(493): 213–219. DOI: 10.1198/jasa.2011. tm10337

Lo, N., D. Griffith, and J.R. Hunter. 1997. "Using a Restricted Adaptive Cluster Sampling to Estimate Pacific Hake Larval Abundance." *California Cooperative Oceanic Fisheries Investigations* 38:103–113.

Low, K.H., G.J. Gordon, J.M. Dolan, and P. Khosla. 2007. "Adaptive Sampling for Multi-Robot Wide-Area Exploration." *Proceedings of the IEEE International Conference on Robotics and Automation*:755–760. Roma, Italy.

Magnussen, S., W. Kurz, D.G. Leckie, and D. Paradine. 2005. "Adaptive Cluster Sampling for Estimation of Deforestation Rates." *European Journal of Forest Research* 124:207–220.

Mohammadi M. 2011. *Nonparametric Confidence Intervals under Adaptive Cluster Sampling*. PhD. Thesis, Department of Mathematical sciences, Isfahan University of Technology, Iran.

Mandallaz, D. 2008. *Sampling Techniques for Forest Inventories*. Boca Raton: Chapman and Hall/CRC.

Muttlak, H.A., and A. Khan. 2002. "Adjusted Two-Stage Adaptive Cluster Sampling." *Environmental and Ecological Statistics* 9:111–120.

Noon, B.R., N.M. Ishwar, and K. Vasudevan. 2006. "Efficiency of Adaptive Cluster and Random Sampling in Detecting Terrestrial Herpetofauna in a Tropical Rainforest." *Wildlife Society Bulletin* 34:59–68.

Ojiambo P.S., and H. Scherm. 2010. "Efficiency of Adaptive Cluster Sampling for Estimating Plant Disease Incidence." *Phytopathology* 100:663–670.

Owen, A.B. 1988. "Empirical Likelihood Confidence Intervals for a Single Functional." *Biometrika* 75:237–249.

Perez, T.D., and J.S. Pontius. 2006. "Conventional Bootstrap and Normal Confidence Interval Estimation under Adaptive Cluster Sampling." *Journal of Statistical Computation and Simulation* 76:755–764.

Philippi, T., 2005. "Adaptive Cluster Sampling for Estimation of Abundances within Local Populations of Low-Abundance Plants." *Ecology* 86:1091–1100.

Pontius, J.A. 1997. "Strip Adaptive Cluster Sampling: Probability Proportional to Size Selection of Primary Units." *Biometrics* 53:1092–1096.

Roesch, F.A. Jr. 1993. "Adaptive Cluster Sampling for Forest Inventories." *Forest Science* 39: 655–669.

Salehi, M.M. 2003. "Comparison Between Hansen-Hurwitz and Horvitz-Thompson Estimators for Adaptive Cluster Sampling." *Environmental and Ecological Statistics*. 10:115–127.

Salehi, M.M. and G.A.F. Seber. 1997. "Adaptive Cluster Sampling with Networks Selected without Replacement." *Biometrika* 84:209–219.

Salehi M.M., and G.A.F. Seber. 2002. "Unbiased Estimators for Restricted Adaptive Cluster Sampling." *Australian and New Zealand Journal of Statistics* 44:63–74.

Salehi, M.M., M. Mohammadi, J.N.K. Rao, and Y.G. Berger. 2010. "Empirical Likelihood Confidence Intervals for Adaptive Cluster Sampling." *Environmental and Ecological Statistics* 17: 111–123.

Särndal, C.E., B. Swensson, and J.H. Wretman. 1992. *Model Assisted Survey Sampling*. New York: Springer-Verlag.

Smith, D.R., J.A. Brown, and N.C.H. Lo. 2004. "Application of Adaptive Cluster Sampling to Biological Populations." In: W.L. Thompson (Ed.) *Sampling Rare and Elusive Species*, 77–122. Washington DC: Island Press.

Smith, D.R., M.J.Conroy, and D.H. Brakhage. 1995. "Efficiency of Adaptive Cluster Sampling for Estimating Density of Wintering Waterfowl." *Biometrics* 51:777–788.

Smith, D.R., B.R. Gray, T.R. Newton, and D. Nichols. 2011. "Effect of Imperfect Detectability on Adaptive and Conventional Sampling: Simulated Sampling of Freshwater Mussels in the Upper Mississippi River." *Environmental Monitoring and Assessment* 170: 499–507. DOI: 10.1007/s10661-009-1251-8.

Smith, D. R., R.F. Villella, and D.P. Lemarie. 2003. "Application of Adaptive Cluster Sampling to Low-Density Populations of Freshwater Mussels." *Environmental and Ecological Statistics* 10:7–15.

St. Clair, K., and D. O'Connell. 2011. "A Bayesian Model for Estimating Population Means Using a Link-Tracing Sampling Design." *Biometrics*, DOI: 10.1111/j.1541-0420.2011.01631.x.

Su, Z., and T.J. Quinn II. 2003. "Estimator Bias and Efficiency for Adaptive Cluster Sampling with Order Statistics and a Stopping Rule." *Environmental and Ecological Statistics* 10(1):17–41.

Sullivan, W.P., B.P. Morrison, and F.W.H. Beamish. 2008. "Adaptive Cluster Sampling: Estimating Density of Spatially Autocorrelated Larvae of the Sea Lamprey with Improved Precision." *Journal of Great Lakes Research* 34:86–97.

Talvitie, M., O. Leino, and M. Holopainen. 2006. "Inventory of Sparse Forest Populations Using Adaptive Cluster Sampling." *Silva Fennica* 40:101–108.

Thompson, S.K. 1990. "Adaptive Cluster Sampling." *Journal of the American Statistical Association* 85:1050–1059.

Thompson, S.K. 1993. "Multivariate Aspects of Adaptive Cluster Sampling." In: G.P. Patil and C.R. Rao (Eds) *Multivariate Environmental Statistics*, 561–572. New York: North Holland/Elsevier Science Publishers.

Thompson, S. K. 1996. "Adaptive Cluster Sampling Based on Order Statistics." *Environmetrics* 7:123–133.

Thompson, S.K. 2006a. "Targeted Random Walk Designs." *Survey Methodology* 32:11–24.

Thompson, S.K. 2006b. "Adaptive Web Sampling." *Biometrics* 62:1224–1234.

Thompson, S.K., and L.M.Collins. 2002. "Adaptive Sampling in Research on Risk-Related Behaviors." *Drug and Alcohol Dependence, Supplement 1* 168: 57–67.

Thompson, S.K., and O. Frank. 2000. "Model-Based Estimation with Link-Tracing Sampling Designs." *Survey Methodology* 26:87–98.

Thompson, S.K., and G.A.F. Seber. 1994. "Detectability in Conventional and Adaptive Sampling." *Biometrics* 50:712–724.

Thompson, S.K., and G.A.F. Seber. 1996. *Adaptive Sampling.* New York: Wiley.

Woodby, D. 1998. "Adaptive Cluster Sampling: Efficiency, Fixed Sample Sizes, and an Application to Red Sea Urchins (Strongylocentrotus Franciscanus) in Southeast Alaska." *Proceedings of the North Pacific Symposium on Invertebrate Stock Assessment and Management* 125:15–20. Canadian special publication of fisheries and aquatic sciences.

Yang, H., C. Kleinn, L. Fehrmann, S. Tang, and S. Magnussen. 2011. A New Design for Sampling with Adaptive Sample Plots. *Environmental and Ecological Statistics* 18:223–237.

Zhang, N., Z. Zhu, and B. Hu. 2000. "On Two-Stage Adaptive Cluster Sampling to Assess Pest Density." *Journal of Zhejiang University* 26:617–620.

Chapter 3
Rao-Blackwell Modifications

Abstract This chapter summarizes some foundational theory for adaptive sampling methods. The Rao-Blackwell theorem can be applied to unbiased estimators to provide more efficient estimators. Closed form expressions for these and related estimators are discussed. The theory is also applied to selecting networks without replacement, and the question of ignoring information from labels is considered.

Keywords Sufficient statistic · Complete statistic · Rao-Blackwell theorem · Adaptive cluster sampling · Networks selected without replacement · Adaptive allocation · Order statistics

3.1 Notation

The theory underlying adaptive sampling from finite populations is more difficult than that associated with infinite populations. We therefore don't propose to consider it in depth as it is developed in detail in Thompson and Seber (1996, Chap. 2). Instead we shall summarize the basic results. To do this we need further notation.

We define $\theta = (y_1, y_2, \ldots, y_N)'$, the unknown population parameter of interest, where $\theta \in \Theta$. All other parameters are functions of θ. We then define an ordered sample of size n as the sequence $s_0 = (i_1, i_2, \ldots, i_n)$ of the labels, some of which may be the same, as in for example sampling with replacement. The data d_0 then consists of the ordered pairs

$$d_0 = ((i_1, y_{i_1}), (i_2, y_{i_2}), \ldots, (i_n, y_{i_n})) = ((i, y_i) : i \in s_0).$$

The notation may be shortened to $d_0 = (s_0, \mathbf{y}_0)$, where $\mathbf{y}_0$ is the set of ordered sample y-values; that is, $\mathbf{y}_0 = (y_i : i \in s_0)$. We shall also be interested in s consisting of the reduced set of ν (= $\nu(s)$) *distinct* labels in s_0, but uniquely ordered from the smallest to the largest label. We define $\mathbf{y}_s$ to be the ordered set of corresponding y-values (in the same order as s). Then, given s_0, we only need $\mathbf{y}_s$ to provide all the information about d_0. To do this we simply match the y-values with the labels in s_0 to

G. A. F. Seber and M. M. Salehi, *Adaptive Sampling Designs*, SpringerBriefs in Statistics,   27
DOI: 10.1007/978-3-642-33657-7_3, © The Author(s) 2013

get $\mathbf{y}_0$. We could therefore redefine d_0 as $d = (s_0, \mathbf{y}_s)$, which in some cases is more convenient. The order of s_0 is usually provided by the order in which the sample is taken, while the reduced sample s is arbitrarily arranged in ascending label order for uniqueness. We will also need the unordered reduced set $s_R = \{i_1, i_2, \ldots, i_\nu\}$ of the ν distinct labels in the sample, and we define $d_R = \{(i, y_i) : i \in s_R\}$. We can express d_R in the form $(s_R, \mathbf{y}_R)$, where $\mathbf{y}_R$ denotes the unordered set of y-values $\{y_{i_1}, y_{i_2}, \ldots, y_{i_\nu}\}$ (that may not be distinct) corresponding to the labels in s_R. In this chapter, random variables will sometimes be denoted by capital letters to avoid confusion so that, for example, D_0 takes the value d_0.

3.2 Sufficiency and Completeness

For reference we give some definitions.[1] The statistic $W = h(D_0)$ is *sufficient* for θ if $P_\theta(D_0 = d_0 \mid W = w)$ is independent of θ for all θ such that $P_\theta(W = w) > 0$. (Here P denotes "probability.") A statistic W_1 is said to be *minimal sufficient* if for every sufficient statistic W there exists a function f such that $W_1 = f(W)$. If f is a one-to-one function, then W is also minimal sufficient. Finally, W is said to be *complete* for θ if for any function $h(W)$, $\mathrm{E}[h(W)] = 0$ for all $\theta \in \Theta$ implies that $h(W) = 0$ with probability 1 for all $\theta \in \Theta$.

We now have the following results from Thompson and Seber (1996).

Theorem 1 Consider an adaptive or conventional design in which the selection probability of the sample does not depend on any of the y-values outside the sample. (The probability may depend on y-values within the sample and may depend on the order of selection.) Then D_R is a minimal sufficient statistic for θ.

Theorem 2 (Rao-Blackwell Theorem) Let $T = T(D_0)$ be any (not necessarily unbiased) estimator of a parameter $\phi = \phi(\theta)$, and let W be sufficient for θ. Define

$$T_W = \mathrm{E}[T \mid W] = \eta(W).$$

Then

1. T_W is an estimator.
2. $\mathrm{E}[T_W] = \mathrm{E}[T]$.
3. If MSE is the Mean-Squared Error, then $\mathrm{MSE}[T_W] \leq \mathrm{MSE}[T]$ with strict inequality for all $\theta \in \Theta$ such that $P_\theta(T \neq T_W) > 0$.
4. If T is unbiased, then mean-squared errors become variances and

$$\mathrm{var}[T_W] = \mathrm{var}[T] - \mathrm{E}_W\{\mathrm{E}(T - T_W)^2 \mid W\}$$
$$= \mathrm{var}[T] - \mathrm{E}_W\{\mathrm{var}[T \mid W]\}.$$

---

[1] These concepts are more difficult for a finite population.

The new estimator T_W is unbiased and has smaller variance provided T is not a function of the minimal sufficient statistic.

Theorem 3 It follows from Theorems 1 and 2 with $W = D_R$ that

$$T_W = T_R = \mathrm{E}[T \mid D_R]$$

is an unbiased estimator with variance at least as small as the variance of T.

For the adaptive designs that follow, the Rao-Blackwell method can be used repeatedly to find practical unbiased estimators. We can start with a simple though perhaps inefficient estimator and then take its conditional expectation given a sufficient statistic to get a better estimator. This raises the question of whether there exists an unbiased estimator of a parameter such as μ that has the smallest variance of all unbiased estimators for all μ, namely the uniformly minimum variance unbiased estimator (UMVUE). This will happen if W is a complete. Unfortunately we have the following result.

Theorem 4 D_R is not complete.

In practice this means that we may be able to derive more than one unbiased estimator that is a function of the minimal sufficient statistic, but one is not uniformly better than any other.

3.3 Rao-Blackwell Applications

We now demonstrate how the above theory can be applied to adaptive cluster sampling (ACS) using a sufficient statistic. We have three unbiased candidates, $\widehat{\mu}_{HT}, \widehat{\mu}_{HH}$, and we can add the obvious inefficient estimator $\overline{y}_1 = \sum_{i=1}^{n_1} y_i$ that only uses the initial selection of units and not any units added adaptively. Since all three estimators depend on the order of selection, as they depend on which n_1 of all the units selected are in the initial sample, they are not functions of D_R. Furthermore the HT and HH estimators do not use all the data information, namely the edge units of the clusters selected. We can therefore apply the Rao-Blackwell theorem to all three estimators.

3.3.1 Adaptive Cluster Sampling

Let T be any one of three estimators, namely the HT and HH estimators and the initial sample mean, with an unbiased estimate of its variance $\widehat{\mathrm{var}}[T]$. Then $T_{RB} = \mathrm{E}[T \mid D_R]$ will be unbiased with smaller variance given by

$$\mathrm{var}[T_{RB}] = \mathrm{var}[T] - \mathrm{E}\{\mathrm{var}[T \mid D_R]\}. \tag{3.1}$$

Let v denote the number of distinct units in the final adaptive sample, and define $G = \binom{v}{n_1}$, the number of possible combinations or "groups" of n_1 distinct units from the v in the sample. Suppose these combinations are indexed in an arbitrary way by the label g ($g = 1, 2, \ldots, G$). Let t_g be the value of T when the initial sample consists of combination g, and let $\widehat{\text{var}}_g[T]$ denote the value of the unbiased estimator $\widehat{\text{var}}[T]$ when computed using the gth combination. We define the indicator variable I_g to be 1 if the gth combination could give rise to d_R (i.e., is compatible with d_R), and 0 otherwise. The number of compatible combinations is then

$$\xi = \sum_{g=1}^{G} I_g$$

and, conditional on d_R, each of these is equally likely. Hence given d_R, $T = t_g$ with probability $1/\xi$ for all compatible g so that

$$T_{RB} = \text{E}[T \mid D_R] = \frac{1}{\xi} \sum_{g=1}^{\xi} t_g = \frac{1}{\xi} \sum_{g=1}^{G} t_g I_g. \tag{3.2}$$

Since $\text{var}[T]$ is also a function θ and $\widehat{\text{var}}[T]$ is an unbiased estimator, we can apply the Rao-Blackwell theorem once again to obtain another unbiased estimator with smaller variance, namely

$$\widehat{\text{var}}_{RB}[T] = \text{E}\{\widehat{\text{var}}[T] \mid D_R\}$$

$$= \frac{1}{\xi} \sum_{g=1}^{\xi} \widehat{\text{var}}_g[T]. \tag{3.3}$$

Also

$$\text{var}[T \mid D_R] = \text{E}[(T - T_{RB})^2 \mid D_R]$$

$$= \frac{1}{\xi} \sum_{g=1}^{\xi} (t_g - T_{RB})^2 \tag{3.4}$$

is an unbiased estimator of its expected value. Combining (3.3) and (3.4) and using (3.1), we get

$$\widehat{\text{var}}[T_{RB}] = \frac{1}{\xi} \sum_{g=1}^{\xi} \{\widehat{\text{var}}_g[T] - (t_g - T_{RB})^2\}$$

$$= \frac{1}{\xi} \sum_{g=1}^{G} \{\widehat{\text{var}}_g[T] - (t_g - T_{RB})^2\} I_g. \tag{3.5}$$

Before applying the above theory to our three estimators we note that $\widehat{\mu}_{HH}$ was based on the frequencies f_i of the number of times that the ith unit appears in the estimator, so we introduce another statistic D_f that consists of D_R together with these frequencies, namely $D_f = \{(i, y_i, f_i) : i \in s_R\}$. One further statistic is of interest, namely $D_J = \{(i, y_i, J_i) : i \in s_R\}$, where J_i is an indicator variable that takes the value 1 when the initial sample intersects the network that contains unit i, and 0 otherwise. From Thompson and Seber (1996, p. 110) and Saheli (2003, p. 118) we have the following results that establish some relationships between the three statistics.

Theorem 5

1. As D_f and D_J are functions of D_R the minimal sufficient statistic (by dropping the f_i and the J_i, respectively), they are sufficient for θ.
2. $\mathrm{E}[\bar{y}_1 \mid D_f] = \widehat{\mu}_{HH}$.
3. $\mathrm{E}[\bar{y}_1 \mid D_R] = \mathrm{E}[\widehat{\mu}_{HH} \mid D_R] (= \widehat{\mu}_{HH,RB})$.
4. $\mathrm{E}[\widehat{\mu}_{HT} \mid D_J] = \widehat{\mu}_{HT}$.

The above results (1) and (2) tell us that when we apply the Rao-Blackwell theorem to both $\bar{y}_1$ and $\widehat{\mu}_{HH}$ we end up with the same estimator $\widehat{\mu}_{HH,RB}$ that will have smaller variance than $\widehat{\mu}_{HH}$. However, from (4), when we condition on the statistic D_J we have no improvement when we apply the Rao-Blackwell theorem to $\widehat{\mu}_{HT}$. On the other hand, Saheli (2003, p. 120) showed that there is an improvement when we apply the theorem to $\widehat{\mu}_{HH}$ conditioning on D_J to get $\tilde{\mu}_{HH}$, say. This indicates that, in some sense, the HT estimator is preferred to the HH estimator. The former has already used all the information in D_J while the latter has not.

We now summarize how we find $\widehat{\mu}_{HT,RB}$ and its unbiased variance estimate. In what follows, the subscript g indicates that computations are carried out using the gth data combination. If ξ is the number of values of g compatible with d_R, we have from Eq. (3.2),

$$\widehat{\mu}_{HT,RB} = \frac{1}{\xi} \sum_{g=1}^{\xi} \widehat{\mu}_{HT,g}$$

and, from (3.5),

$$\widehat{\mathrm{var}}[\widehat{\mu}_{HT,RB}] = \frac{1}{\xi} \sum_{g=1}^{\xi} \{\widehat{\mathrm{var}}_g[\widehat{\mu}_{HT}] - (\widehat{\mu}_{HT,g} - \widehat{\mu}_{HT,RB})^2\}.$$

To obtain similar results for the HH estimator we simply replace HT by HH in the above expressions to get $\widehat{\mu}_{HH,RB}$ and its variance estimator. Substantial computations are required to obtain ξ and to compute expressions for each of the g combinations compatible with D_R. More helpful formulae are needed. For example, Salehi (1999) introduced closed forms for both $\widehat{\mu}_{HH,RB}$ and $\widehat{\mu}_{HT,RB}$ along with unbiased estimators of their variances using the "inclusion–exclusion" formula which can be more readily computed. He illustrated his computations, notation, and conclusions via a small population example and an analysis of a set of data from Smith et al. (1995). For the latter, he deliberately selected an initial sample demanding the most computation. In both examples, $\widehat{\mu}_{HH,RB}$ was more efficient than $\widehat{\mu}_{HT,RB}$. Even though these results suggested otherwise, Thompson and Seber (1996, p. 111) mentioned that neither $\widehat{\mu}_{HH,RB}$ nor $\widehat{\mu}_{HT,RB}$ is uniformly better than the other (see also Turk and Borkowski 2005).

Felix-Medina (2000) derived closed-form expressions of Rao-Blackwell modified HT estimators for ACS with an initial simple random sample and for ACS with an initial unequal probability sample with replacement. Expressions for the variances of these estimators, as well as closed-forms for unbiased Rao-Blackwell estimators of those variances, were also derived. Derivations were based on the multivariate hypergeometric distribution for ACS. These closed-forms allow users of ACS to take advantage of computer software that compute probabilities from the hypergeometric distribution.

Low et al. (2005) implemented the ACS design for multi-robot wide area prospecting. Robots could exploit the clustering nature of the environmental phenomena (i.e., hotspots) and therefore perform better than simple random sampling and systematic sampling in such environments. Quantitative experimental results in the simulation of the mineral prospecting task showed that the ACS design was the most efficient in exploration by yielding more minerals and information with fewer resources. Low et al. used Salehi's closed form formulas for $\widehat{\mu}_{HH,RB}$ and $\widehat{\mu}_{HT,RB}$ to evaluate the Rao-Blackwellized estimators. Their results showed that these estimators also provided more efficient mineral density estimates than the estimators using other sampling methods. In their study, $\widehat{\mu}_{HT,RB}$ was more efficient than $\widehat{\mu}_{HH,RB}$.

Low et al. (2005) commented that since (3.2) and (3.5) are based on compatible sample sets, the ξ compatible samples have to be identified from the G combinations and their corresponding ξ estimators have to be evaluated. Here ξ and G can be potentially large, which would render the Rao-Blackwellized method computationally difficult. However, closed-form expressions exist for the Rao-Blackwellized estimators. These expressions are computationally efficient if relatively few networks of size larger than 1 are intersected by the initial sample. This assumption is valid if the prospecting region contains only a few hotspots. It is therefore sensible to look at an intermediate solution. Dryver and Thompson (2005) derived two easy-to-compute estimators of higher efficiency than their corresponding original estimators $\widehat{\mu}_{HT}$ and $\widehat{\mu}_{HT}$ by taking the expected value of the usual estimators conditional on a sufficient statistic that is not minimally sufficient. They incorporated only those edge units that were in the initial sample.

Deriving Rao-Blackwell versions of the HT and HH estimators of a ratio (see Salehi 2001) or of the ratio estimators (see Dryver and Chao 2007) for ACS is much more complicated. Chao et al. (2011) noted that the approaches used by Salehi (1999) and Felix-Medina (2000) do not provide simplified analytical forms of their Rao-Blackwellized versions. They proposed four alternative improved ratio estimators in which the Rao-Blackwellization technique is utilized in a straightforward manner. By dropping the population mean of the auxiliary variable from the proposed estimators one can readily have improved estimators of a ratio.

3.3.2 Selecting Networks Without Replacement

Adaptive cluster sampling with networks selected without replacement was discussed in Sect. 2.4. We recall the following estimates:

$$\widehat{\mu}_M = \frac{1}{N} \sum_{i=1}^{n} \frac{P(s_R \mid i)}{P(s_R)} y_i^*, \tag{3.6}$$

where y_i^* is the sum of the y values in the ith network, and unbiased variance estimate

$$\widehat{\mathrm{var}}[\widehat{\mu}_M] = \frac{1}{N^2} \sum_{i=1}^{n} \sum_{j<i}^{n} x_i x_j \left(\frac{P(s_R \mid i, j)}{P(s_R)} - \frac{P(s_R \mid i) P(s_R \mid j)}{P(s_R)^2} \right) (w_i - w_j)^2, \tag{3.7}$$

where $w_i = y_i^*/x_i$ is the mean of the y values in the ith network. As we don't use some information from edge units, we can improve on the above estimates using the Rao-Blackwell theorem.

Following Salehi and Seber (1997), we have ν distinct networks in the final sample of which n are initially selected. The difference $\nu - n$ consists of the edge units (networks of size one) that are part of the clusters but are not part of the initial sample. Let $d_R = \{(i_1, y_{i_1}^*), \ldots, (i_\nu, y_{i_\nu}^*)\}$ represent the final unordered sample of the ν distinct networks with their labels; ν is now random. Applying the above theory to networks rather than units we have that for any adaptive sampling scheme, D_R is a minimal sufficient statistic for $(y_1^*, y_2^*, \ldots, y_K^*)$. Since $\widehat{\mu}_M$ is not a function of d_R as it does not use any of the $(\nu - n)$ edge units added adaptively and not selected in the initial sample, we can use the Rao-Blackwell theorem to improve on our estimate as follows.

Suppose there are h edge units in the final sample, that is in d_R, then $h - (\nu - n)$ of these are initially selected as networks of size one not satisfying the condition C and are successively "removed" from the population, but are later found to be among the edge units of the initially selected clusters. Let s_g be the subset of size n of d_R which, when taken as the initial sample of networks, leads to d_R, and let $\widehat{\mu}_{M,g}$ be Murthy's estimator associated with s_g. To specify the number of such subsets we must have all the $(\nu - h)$ non-edge units belong to s_g: we denote this part of s_g by $s_{(1)}$. To add to $s_{(1)}$ to make up s_g we can choose $\{n - (\nu - h)\}$ of the h edge units in d_R which can be done in

$$G_h = \binom{h}{n - (\nu - h)}$$

ways. If $s_{(2)g}$ represents one of these subsets, then s_g is made up of $s_{(1)}$ and $s_{(2)g}$ ($g = 1, 2, \ldots, G_h$). The Rao-Blackwell estimator is given by

$$\widehat{\mu}_{RB} = E[\widehat{\mu}_M \mid D_R = d_R] = \frac{1}{G_h} \sum_{g=1}^{G_h} \widehat{\mu}_{M,g} = \frac{1}{N G_h} \sum_{g=1}^{G_h} \sum_{i \in s_g} \frac{P(s_g \mid i)}{P(s_g)} y_i^*.$$

Since all the s_g contain $s_{(1)}$, and the networks corresponding to edge units contain just one unit, $P(s_g \mid i)/P(s_g)$ has a common a value for all g that we denote by $P(s \mid i)/P(s)$, where s is the initial sample of n networks. Since each of the networks in each $s_{(2)g}$ contains just one unit, $P(s \mid i)$ is the same for all i so we can denote it by $P(s \mid i_1)$, say. Then

$$
\hat{\mu}_{RB} = \frac{1}{NG_h} \sum_{g=1}^{G_h} \sum_{i \in s_{(1)}} \frac{P(s \mid i)}{P(s)} y_i^* + \frac{1}{NG_h} \sum_{g=1}^{G_h} \sum_{i \in s_{(2)g}} \frac{P(s \mid i_1)}{P(s)} y_i^*
$$

$$
= \frac{1}{N} \sum_{i \in s_{(1)}} \frac{P(s \mid i)}{P(s)} y_i^* + \frac{P(s \mid i_1)}{P(s)} \frac{1}{NG_h} \sum_{g=1}^{G_h} \sum_{i \in s_{(2)g}} y_i^* .
$$

For simplicity we let the networks in d_R be indexed as $i = 1, 2, \ldots, v - h$, and those corresponding to edge units indexed as $i = v - h + 1, \ldots, v$. Since the number of times a particular y_i^* appears in the second double summation is G_{h-1}, we have

$$
\hat{\mu}_{RB} = \sum_{i=1}^{v-h} \frac{P(s \mid i)}{NP(s)} y_i^* + \frac{P(s \mid i_1)}{NP(s)} \frac{G_{h-1}}{G_h} \sum_{i=v-h+1}^{v} y_i^*
$$

$$
= \sum_{i=1}^{v-h} \frac{P(s \mid i)}{NP(s)} y_i^* + \frac{P(s \mid i_1)}{NP(s)} \{n - (v - h)\} \bar{y}_e ,
$$

where $\bar{y}_e$ is the mean of the h edge units in d_R. We know from (3.1) that

$$
\mathrm{var}[\hat{\mu}_{RB}] = \mathrm{var}[\hat{\mu}_M] - \mathrm{E}\{\mathrm{var}[\hat{\mu}_M \mid d_R]\},
$$

and Saheli and Seber (1997, pp. 213–214) proved that an unbiased estimator of the above variance is

$$
\widehat{\mathrm{var}}[\hat{\mu}_{RB}] = \frac{1}{G_h} \sum_{g=1}^{G_h} \widehat{\mathrm{var}}_g[\hat{\mu}_M] - \left\{ \frac{P(s \mid i_1)}{NP(s)} \right\}^2 \{n - (v - h)\}^2 s_e^2 ,
$$

where

$$
s_e^2 = \frac{1}{G_h} \sum_{i=1}^{G_h} (\bar{y}_g^* - \bar{y}_e)^2 , \qquad \bar{y}_g^* = \frac{1}{n - (v - h)} \sum_{i \in s_{s(2)g}} y_i^* ,
$$

and $\widehat{\mathrm{var}}_g[\hat{\mu}_M]$ is Eq. (3.7) applied to s_g. They also give a small numerical example of the method.

3.4 Ignoring the Labels

In Chap. 6, where we consider adaptive allocation, we don't focus on adaptive cluster sampling as it is the allocation that is adaptive. There are sampling situations such as simple random sampling (SRS) when we don't need to use the labels. In fact it is the use of the labels in D_R that leads to Theorem 4 and the lack of completeness. Assuming SRS and using the notation of Sect. 3.2, we have $\nu = n$ and $\mathbf{y}_R$ is the unordered set of (not necessarily distinct) y-values. We define $\mathbf{y}_{rank} = (y_{(1)}, y_{(2)}, \ldots, y_{(n)})$ to be the set of y's in $\mathbf{y}_R$ ranked according to size, namely $y_{(1)} \leq y_{(2)} \leq \cdots, y_{(n)}$. We note that the reduced set $\mathbf{y}_R$ and the order statistics $\mathbf{y}_{rank}$ are equivalent in the sense that the knowledge of one implies knowledge of the other. Let V be a subset of $\mathbb{R}$ and define Θ to be the Cartesian product

$$\Theta = V \times V \times \cdots \times V = \mathbb{R}^N(V), \quad \text{say.}$$

We then have the following theorem (Thompson and Seber 1996, pp. 47–48).

Theorem 6 The order statistics $\mathbf{y}_{rank}$ are complete for θ when $\theta \in \Theta = \mathbb{R}^N(V)$.

In applying this theorem we assume that s_R is unknown or knowledge of s_R is discarded from D_R. The labels are only used to carry out a particular sampling design. We shall use the above theorem in Chap. 6.

References

Chao C-T., A.L. Dryver, and T.C. Chiang. 2011. "Leveraging the Rao-Blackwell Theorem to Improve Ratio Estimators in Adaptive Cluster sampling." *Environmental and Ecological Statistics* DOI:10.1007/s10651-010-0151-y.

Dryver, A.L., and C-T. Chao. 2007. "Ratio Estimators in Adaptive Cluster Sampling." *Environmetrics* 18:607–620.

Dryver, A.L., and S.K. Thompson. 2005. "Improved Unbiased Estimators in Adaptive Cluster Sampling." *Journal of the Royal Statistical Society* 67(1):157–166.

Félix-Medina, M.H. 2000. "Analytical Expressions for Rao-Blackwell Estimators in Adaptive Cluster Sampling." *Journal of Statistical Planning and Inference* 84:221–236.

Low K.H., G.J. Gordon, J.M. Dolan, and P. Khosla. 2005. "Adaptive Sampling for Multi-Robot Wide Area Prospecting." Robotics Institute, CMU, Pittsburgh, PA, Tech. Rep. CMU-RI-TR-05-51. (See http://citeseer.ist.psu.edu/viewdoc/summary?doi=10.1.1.72.4649.)

Salehi M.M. 1999. "Rao-Blackwell Versions of the Horvitz-Thompson and Hansen-Hurwitz Estimators in Adaptive Cluster Sampling." *Journal of Environmental and Ecological Statistics* 6:183–195.

Salehi M.M. 2001. "Application of Adaptive Sampling in Fishery, Part 1: Adaptive Cluster Sampling and Its Strip Versions." *Iranian Journal of Fisheries Sciences* 3(1):55–76.

Salehi M. M. 2003. "Comparison Between Hansen-Hurwitz and Horvitz- Estimators for Adaptive Cluster Sampling." *Journal of Environmental and Ecological Statistics* 10(1):115–127.

Salehi M. M., and G.A.F. Seber. 1997. "Adaptive Cluster Sampling Design with the Networks Selected without Replacement." *Biometrika* 84:209–219.

Smith, D. R., M.J. Conroy, and D.H. Brakhage. 1995. "Efficiency of Adaptive Cluster Sampling
   for Estimating Density of Wintering Waterfowl." *Biometrics* 51:777–788.
Thompson, S.K., and G.A.F. Seber. 1996. *Adaptive Sampling*. New York: Wiley.
Turk, P., and J.J. Borkowski. 2005. "A Review of Adaptive Cluster Sampling: 1990–2003." *Environmental and Ecological Statistics* 12:55–94.

Chapter 4
Primary and Secondary Units

Abstract In adaptive sampling, the sampling units can sometimes be divided into primary and secondary units. After a sample of primary units is taken, adaptive cluster sampling can be carried out within each primary unit selected using either a sample or all of its secondary units. Primary units can be a variety of shapes such as strip transects or Latin squares. Two procedures are possible depending on whether adaptive clusters are allowed to cross primary unit boundaries or not. Stratified sampling is a special case in which all the primary units or strata are sampled. Two stage-sampling can be used for carrying out a pilot survey to determine how to design a full-scale survey.

Keywords Primary units · Two-stage adaptive sampling · Stratified adaptive sampling · Design an adaptive survey

4.1 Introduction

In some surveys of natural or human populations it is more convenient to group the units (referred to here as secondary units) into larger units called primary units, and then sample these first. For example, if the population is a rectangle, it can be divided up into equal-width strips as primary units running the full length of the population area. In its adaptive modification each strip is divided up into smaller secondary units of the same size. We sample *all* the secondary units in a chosen primary unit and, if condition $C(y_i > c)$ is satisfied for any secondary unit, we then sample adaptively in the neighborhood of the unit (say a "cross" of units). This gives us a cluster of units, as before, which can overlap with other primary units. Unit (i, j), the jth secondary unit in the ith primary unit, is said to satisfy the condition of interest C if y_{ij} is in a specified set such as defined by $y_{ij} > c$ (often $c = 0$).

Strip transects have been widely used, for example, in aerial and ship surveys of animals and marine mammals. The aircraft (airplane or helicopter) or vessel travels down a line and the area is surveyed on either side out to a given distance. Also used are line transects that are divided up into shorter transects (secondary units).

G. A. F. Seber and M. M. Salehi, *Adaptive Sampling Designs*, SpringerBriefs in Statistics,   37
DOI: 10.1007/978-3-642-33657-7_4, © The Author(s) 2013

Here the adaptive part of the sampling relates to the intensity of the sampling effort (Pollard et al. 2002). Thompson (1991a) introduced the idea of primary and secondary units for adaptive cluster sampling and his theory from Thompson and Seber (1996, Sect. 4.7) is now given.

4.2 Simple Random Sample of Primary Units

Suppose we have N primary units each consisting of M secondary units. The population parameters of interest are

$$\tau = \sum_{i=1}^{N} \sum_{j=1}^{M} y_{ij} \text{ and } \mu = \tau/MN.$$

As before, we divide up the population of MN secondary units into K distinct networks using clusters without their edge units. We define y_k^* to be the sum of the y-values in the kth network ($k = 1, 2, \ldots, K$), and now x_k denotes the number of *primary* units in the population that intersect the kth network. Suppose that we take a simple random sample of n_1 primary units and then sample all the secondary units in the primary unit with adaptive additions that cross primary unit boundaries. We define J_k to take the value of 1 with (intersection) probability α_k if the initial sample of primary units intersects the kth network, and 0 otherwise. The HT estimator is again given by Eq. (2.7), namely

$$\widehat{\mu}_{\mathrm{HT}} = \frac{1}{MN} \sum_{i=1}^{K} \frac{y_k^* J_k}{\alpha_k} = \frac{1}{MN} \sum_{k=1}^{\kappa} \frac{y_k^*}{\alpha_k}, \tag{4.1}$$

where N is replaced by MN, κ is the number of distinct networks in the sample, and α_k is given by Eq. (2.8). Using the same argument that led to Eq. (2.9), we have

$$\alpha_{rs} = 1 - \left[\binom{N - x_r}{n_1} + \binom{N - x_s}{n_1} - \binom{N - x_r - x_s + x_{rs}}{n_1} \right] \Big/ \binom{N}{n_1},$$

where α_{rs} is the probability that the initial sample of primary units intersects both networks r and s, and x_{rs} is the number of primary units that intersect both networks. The variance of $\widehat{\mu}_{HT}$ and it unbiased estimator are given by Eqs. (2.10) and (2.11), but with N replaced by MN, namely

$$\mathrm{var}[\widehat{\mu}_{HT}] = \frac{1}{M^2 N^2} \left[\sum_{j=1}^{K} \sum_{k=1}^{K} y_j^* y_k^* \left(\frac{\alpha_{jk} - \alpha_j \alpha_k}{\alpha_j \alpha_k} \right) \right], \tag{4.2}$$

with an unbiased estimate

$$\widehat{\text{var}}[\widehat{\mu}_{HT}] = \frac{1}{M^2 N^2} \left[\sum_{j=1}^{K} \sum_{k=1}^{K} y_j^* y_k^* \left(\frac{\alpha_{jk} - \alpha_j \alpha_k}{\alpha_{jk} \alpha_j \alpha_k} \right) J_j J_k \right]$$

$$= \frac{1}{M^2 N^2} \left[\sum_{j=1}^{K} \sum_{k=1}^{K} \frac{y_j^* y_k^*}{\alpha_{jk}} \left(\frac{\alpha_{jk}}{\alpha_j \alpha_k} - 1 \right) \right], \qquad (4.3)$$

where α_{jj} is interpreted as α_j.

If b_k is the number of times network k is intersected by the initial sample of primary networks, we can also use the HH estimator from Eq. (2.17), namely

$$\widehat{\mu}_{HH} = \frac{1}{MN} \sum_{k=1}^{K} y_k^* \frac{b_k}{E[b_k]},$$

$$= \frac{1}{Mn_1} \sum_{k=1}^{K} \frac{b_k y_k^*}{x_k},$$

since b_k has the hypergeometric distribution with parameters (N, x_k, n_1) and mean $n_1 x_k / N$. We note that

$$b_k = \sum_{i=1}^{n_1} J_{ik},$$

where $J_{ik} = 1$ if the ith primary unit intersects the kth network, and 0 otherwise. Hence

$$\widehat{\mu}_{HH} = \frac{1}{n_1 M} \sum_{i=1}^{n_1} \sum_{k=1}^{K} \frac{J_{ik} y_k^*}{x_k}$$

$$= \frac{1}{n_1} \sum_{i=1}^{n_1} w_i$$

$$= \overline{w}, \qquad (4.4)$$

where

$$w_i = \frac{1}{M} \sum_{k=1}^{K} \frac{J_{ik} y_k^*}{x_k} = \frac{1}{M} \sum_{k=1}^{\kappa_i} \frac{y_k^*}{x_k},$$

and κ_i is the number of networks that intersect the ith primary unit. From Eqs. (2.15) and (2.16) we have

$$\text{var}[\widehat{\mu}_{HH}] = \frac{N - n_1}{Nn_1(N-1)} \sum_{i=1}^{N}(w_i - \mu)^2,$$

with unbiased estimate

$$\widehat{\text{var}}[\widehat{\mu}_{HH}] = \frac{N - n_1}{Nn_1(n_1-1)} \sum_{i=1}^{n_1}(w_i - \widehat{\mu}_{HH})^2.$$

4.3 Other Primary Units

Other shapes are possible for the primary units. For example, a single primary unit may consist of a collection of small same-shaped clusters of secondary units spaced systematically throughout the population area instead of being contiguous (all together). One then chooses the primary units systematically but using a random starting point. Unfortunately we don't get unbiased estimation of the variance. Munholland and Borkowski (1993, 1996) and Borkowski (1999) suggested using a Latin square +1 design selected from a square grid of secondary units. The Latin square gives a secondary unit in every row and column of the grid, and the extra (i.e. +1) unit ensures that any pair of units has a positive probability of being included in the initial sample. The latter requirement is needed for unbiased variance estimation. It essentially combines the features of a systematic sample with additional random sampling and allows for unbiased estimation of the variance using a HT estimator. It can be regarded as a type of "space-filling" design. For some details and examples see Thompson (1991a) and Thompson and Seber (1996, pp. 128–134). There are two major restrictions for the simple Latin square design +1: (i) populations units must be arranged in a square and (ii) the sample size must be $N + 1$ from a population of size N^2. Borkowski (2003) introduced a class of sampling designs called Simple Latin Square Sampling $\pm k$ that reasonably deals with restriction (ii) as they have the flexibility to allow for different sample sizes. Salehi (2006) introduced a row and column elimination sampling design that deals with both restrictions. Hung (2011) introduced an adaptive version of a space-filling design called the probability-based Latin hypercube design.

Adaptive cluster sampling has greater efficiency and higher probabilities of observing rare events for a rare and clustered population when the initial sampling has a good coverage of the population area. Acharya et al. (2000) used systematic adaptive cluster sampling to assess rare tree species. The tree species under study were found in clusters, and they concluded that efficiency of adaptive sampling depended on cluster size, with greatest efficiency observed for the species that formed the largest clusters. Salehi (2004) proved that optimal sampling under a spatial correlation model for any population of units arranged in a rectangle will be a combination of systematic and Latin square sampling whenever the optimal design exists. Salehi (2002) suggested using a systematic Latin square sampling +1 design selected from a rectangular grid of secondary units.

Félix-Medina and Thompson (2004) presented a multi-phase variant of adaptive cluster sampling that allows the sampler to control the number of measurements of the variable of interest. A first-phase sample is selected using an adaptive cluster sampling design based on an easy-to-measure auxiliary variable that is correlated with the variable of interest. The network structure of the adaptive cluster sample is used to select either an ordinary one-phase or two-phase subsample of units. They estimated the population mean by either a regression-type estimator or a Horvitz-Thompson-type estimator. The results of their simulation study showed a good performance of the proposed design.

4.4 Two-Stage Adaptive Cluster Sampling

This design is similar to the simple random sample of primary units described in Sect. 4.2 except that after the initial selection of the primary units we don't sample all the units in each selected primary unit. Instead we take a simple random sample of primary sampling units (PSUs) as before, but then take a subsample of secondary units within each of the selected PSUs and add adaptively. We then have the choice of two designs. As we add secondary units adaptively we can either stop at the boundary of the PSU or allow overlap into neighboring PSUs. We focus on this method as it also provides one way of carrying out a pilot survey that can be used to design a full survey to achieve a given accuracy.

4.4.1 Notation

Suppose that we have a total population of N_T secondary units that are partitioned into M primary units of size N_i units ($i = 1, 2, \ldots, M$). Usually we endeavor to have all the N_i the same. Let the unit (i, j) denote the jth unit in the ith primary unit with an associated measurement or count y_{ij}. Let $\tau_i = \sum_{j=1}^{N_i} y_{ij}$ be the sum of the y-values in the ith primary unit, and let $\tau = \sum_{i=1}^{M} \tau_i$ be the total for the whole population. The population mean per unit is then given by $\mu = \tau/N_T$. In the first stage of the sampling, we choose a simple random sample of m of the M primary units without replacement, though this requirement of simple random sampling can be relaxed in some situations, as we shall see later. At the second stage, we take an initial simple random sample of n_i secondary units without replacement from primary unit i ($i = 1, 2, \ldots, M$) so that $n_0 = \sum_{i=1}^{m} n_i$ is the total initial sample size.

4.4.2 Overlapping Scheme

Ignoring PSU boundaries, suppose that the N_T units are partitioned into K networks by the condition C and the type of neighborhood used. Once again we can use our usual HT estimator without the edge units, namely,

$$\widehat{\mu}_{HT} = \frac{1}{N_T} \sum_{k=1}^{K} \frac{y_k^* J_k}{\alpha_k}, \tag{4.5}$$

where the K distinct networks are labeled $1, 2, \ldots, K$ regardless of primary boundaries, J_k is an indicator variable taking the value 1 (with probability α_k, say) if the initial sample of size n_0 intersects network k (i.e., contains at least one unit from the network k) and 0 otherwise, and y_k^* is the usual sum of the y-values for network k. We obtain the variance of $\widehat{\mu}_{HT}$ and its estimate from Eqs. (4.2) and (4.3) by replacing MN by N_T. Expressions for the α_i and α_{rs} are complex and are given in the Appendix of Salehi and Seber (1997). Also an HH-type estimator is derived in that paper.

4.4.3 Non-Overlapping Scheme

When the clusters are truncated at primary unit boundaries, each primary unit can be treated separately. Thus if the ith primary unit is selected, an unbiased estimate of that unit's total y-value is $\widehat{\tau}_i = \sum_{k=1}^{K_i} y_{ik}^* J_{ik} / \alpha_{ik}$, where K_i is the number of networks in the primary unit i, y_{ik}^* is the sum of the y-values associated with network k, and α_{ik} ($= \mathrm{E}[J_k]$) is the probability that the initial sample of units in primary unit i intersects network k. If x_{ik} is the number of units in network k that are located in primary unit i, then

$$\alpha_{ik} = 1 - \binom{N_i - x_{ik}}{n_i} \bigg/ \binom{N_i}{n_i}. \tag{4.6}$$

From the theory of sampling without replacement, an unbiased "estimator" of $\sum_{i=1}^{M} \tau_i / M$ is $\sum_{i=1}^{m} \tau_i / m$ so that replacing τ_i by $\widehat{\tau}_i$, an estimate of the overall mean is

$$\widehat{\mu}_1 = \frac{1}{N_T} M \sum_{i=1}^{m} \frac{\widehat{\tau}_i}{m} = \frac{M\overline{w}}{N_T}, \text{ say,} \tag{4.7}$$

where $w_i = \widehat{\tau}_i$. To find its variance, we need the probability that the initial sample of units in primary unit i intersects both the r and s networks, namely [c.f. Eq. (2.9)]

$$\alpha_{irs} = \alpha_{ir} + \alpha_{is} - \left[1 - \binom{N_i - x_{ir} - x_{is}}{n_i} \bigg/ \binom{N_i}{n_i} \right]. \tag{4.8}$$

Also, from Eq. (4.2),

$$V_i = \text{var}[\widehat{\tau}_i] = \sum_{r=1}^{K_i} \sum_{s=1}^{K_i} y_{ir}^* y_{is}^* \left(\frac{\alpha_{irs} - \alpha_{ir}\alpha_{is}}{\alpha_{ir}\alpha_s} \right).$$

Applying the theory of two-stage sampling from Särndal, Swensson, and Wretman (1992, p.137) to the sample mean $\overline{w}$, Salehi and Seber (1997) showed that

$$\text{var}[\widehat{\mu}_1] = \frac{1}{N_T^2} M(M-m) \frac{\sigma_M^2}{m} + \frac{1}{N_T^2} \frac{M}{m} \sum_{i=1}^{M} V_i, \tag{4.9}$$

where

$$\sigma_M^2 = \frac{1}{M-1} \sum_{i=1}^{M} (\tau_i - \overline{\tau})^2 \quad \text{and} \quad \overline{\tau} = \frac{1}{M} \sum_{i=1}^{M} \tau_i.$$

An unbiased estimate of the above variance is

$$\widehat{\text{var}}[\widehat{\mu}_1] = \frac{1}{N_T^2} M(M-m) \frac{s_M^2}{m} + \frac{1}{N_T^2} \frac{M}{m} \sum_{i=1}^{m} \widehat{V}_i, \tag{4.10}$$

where

$$s_M^2 = \frac{1}{m-1} \sum_{i=1}^{m} (\widehat{\tau}_i - \frac{1}{m} \sum_{i=1}^{m} \widehat{\tau}_i)^2, \tag{4.11}$$

and

$$\widehat{V}_i = \sum_{r=1}^{\kappa_i} \sum_{s=1}^{\kappa_i} y_{ir}^* y_{is}^* \left(\frac{\alpha_{irs} - \alpha_{ir}\alpha_{is}}{\alpha_{irs}\alpha_{ir}\alpha_{is}} \right). \tag{4.12}$$

Here κ_i is the number of distinct networks intersected in primary unit i. As the distinct unordered units and their labels form a minimal sufficient statistic for any adaptive sampling scheme, the Rao-Blackwell theorem can be used to provide unbiased estimators with smaller variances. For example, the estimators $\widehat{\tau}_i$ in $\widehat{\mu}_1$ can be replaced by their Rao-Blackwell versions.

An HH estimator can also be derived and details are given briefly by Salehi and Seber (1997). The HT $\widehat{\mu}_1$ estimator seems to be preferred for a number of reasons, such as better efficiency in many situations. It can be also used, for the non-overlapping case, to design such an experiment using a pilot survey, which we now consider briefly. One disadvantage of this estimator is that individual PSU variance estimates $\widehat{V}_i$ in (4.12) may be negative. If constant n_i is used, we recommend keeping n_i small. If $n_i = 2$, then it is shown in Appendix 3 of Salehi and Seber (1997) that $\widehat{V}_i$ is always nonnegative. Finally we note that Rocco (2008) proposed a restricted version of two-stage adaptive cluster sampling, adopting a similar approach to Salehi and Seber (2002).

4.4.4 Pilot Survey

It transpires that when m/M is small (say less then 0.1) the second term of (4.9) is generally negligible (Särndal et al. 1992, p. 139) and $\text{var}[\widehat{\mu}_1] < v$, where

$$v = \text{E}\left(\frac{M^2 s_M^2}{N_T^2 m}\right).$$

Suppose that a pilot survey has been run in which a sample of size m_0 PSUs has been chosen and the n_i are selected according to the same rules to be used for the full survey being planned. From the pilot survey, we can use the formula for s_M^2 but with m_0 instead of m to get s_0^2, say, which can be shown to have the same expected value as s_M^2. Then the number of PSUs that we need to sample in the full survey to achieve a desired value of v is approximately given by

$$m = \frac{M^2 s_0^2}{N_T^2 v}.$$

Cost considerations can also be taken into account as in Salehi and Seber (1997), who also gave an example demonstrating the calculations.

4.5 Stratified Adaptive Cluster Sampling

If we happen to know some prior information about where aggregations are likely to occur we can use stratification to reduce some of the variability in the estimators. Christman (2000) suggests that the best form of stratification is when rare objects are in a single small stratum that is disproportionately oversampled. In stratified sampling each stratum is like a primary unit and all primary units are selected. Once again we have two scenarios depending on whether we allow overlapping of stratum boundaries or not. We assume simple random sampling in each stratum. This theory is based on Thompson (1991b) and also given by Thompson and Seber (1996, Sect. 4.9).

4.5.1 Overlapping Strata

Suppose the total population of N units is partitioned into H strata, with N_h units in the hth stratum ($h = 1, 2, \ldots, H$). Define unit (h, i) to be the ith unit in the hth stratum with associated y-value y_{hi}. A simple random sample of n_h units is taken from the hth stratum so that $n_0 = \sum_{h=1}^{H} n_h$ is the initial total sample size. Further units are added adaptively without regard to stratum boundaries. Ignoring the edge units, we then have the usual HT estimator [cf. (4.5)] and, using the same notation,

$$\widehat{\mu}_{HT,st} = \frac{1}{N_T} \sum_{k=1}^{K} \frac{y_k^* J_k}{\alpha_k},$$

with α_k, the probability of intersecting network k with initial samples in each of the strata, is now given by

$$\alpha_k = 1 - \prod_{h=1}^{H} \left[\binom{N_h - x_{hk}}{n_k} \Big/ \binom{N_h}{n_h} \right],$$

where x_{hk} is the number of units in stratum h that lie in network k. This will be zero if network k lies totally outside stratum h. If the network straddles a boundary, then we ignore the network units that lie outside stratum h in the definition of x_{hk}. Since $E[J_k] = \alpha_k$, $\widehat{\mu}_{HH,st}$ is unbiased. To find its variance we need α_{rs}, the probability that the initial sample intersects both networks r and s, namely [cf. (2.9)]

$$\alpha_{rs} = 1 - (1 - \alpha_r) - (1 - \alpha_s) + \prod_{h=1}^{H} \left[\binom{N_h - x_{hr} - x_{hs}}{n_h} \Big/ \binom{N_h}{n_h} \right].$$

Its variance and unbiased estimate are given by Eqs. (2.10) and (2.11).

We now consider an HH-type estimator based on the numbers of initial intersections. To do this we define A_{hi} to be the network containing unit (h, i), and A_{ghi}, that part of A_{hi} in stratum g. Let f_{ghi} be the number of units from the initial sample in stratum g that fall in A_{ghi}, and let m_{ghi} be the number of units in A_{ghi}. Then

$$f_{\cdot hi} = \sum_{g=1}^{H} f_{ghi}$$

is the number of units from the initial sample of n_0 units that fall in A_{hi}. This will be zero if no initial units in the hth stratum intersect A_{hi}. Equation (2.13) now translates into

$$\widehat{\mu}_{HH,st} = \frac{1}{N} \sum_{h=1}^{H} \sum_{i=1}^{N_h} y_{hi} \frac{f_{\cdot hi}}{E[f_{\cdot hi}]},$$

which is unbiased. Since f_{ghi} has a hypergeometric distribution with parameters (N_g, m_{ghi}, n_g), $E[f_{ghi}] = n_g m_{ghi}/N_g$ and

$$E[f_{\cdot hi}] = \sum_{g=1}^{H} \frac{n_g}{N_g} m_{ghi}.$$

To find $\mathrm{var}[\widehat{\mu}_{HH,st}]$, we express $\widehat{\mu}_{HH,st}$ in terms of weighted means. The term $y_{hi} f_{\cdot hi}$ tells us that A_{hi} is intersected $f_{\cdot hi}$ times so that $\widehat{\mu}_{HH,st}$ is the weighted sum of all the units eventually sampled, with some networks repeated. Also, the weight $\mathrm{E}[f_{\cdot hi}]$ is the same for each unit in A_{hi}. If Y_{hi} is the sum of the y-values in A_{hi}, then

$$\widehat{\mu}_{HH,st} = \frac{1}{N} \sum_{h=1}^{H} \sum_{i=1}^{n_h} \frac{Y_{hi}}{\mathrm{E}[f_{\cdot hi}]},$$

$$= \sum_{h=1}^{H} \frac{N_h}{N} \overline{w}_h, \tag{4.13}$$

where

$$\overline{w}_h = \frac{1}{n_h} \sum_{i=1}^{n_h} w_{hi} \quad \text{and} \quad w_{hi} = \frac{n_h}{N_h} \cdot \frac{Y_{hi}}{\mathrm{E}[f_{\cdot hi}]}.$$

We see that (4.13) takes the form of a stratified sample mean of a stratified random sample taken without replacement in which the variable of interest is w_{hi}. The stratum mean and variance for this variable are

$$\overline{W}_h = \frac{1}{N_h} \sum_{i=1}^{N_h} w_{hi} \quad \text{and} \quad \sigma_h^2 = \frac{1}{N_h - 1} \sum_{i=1}^{N_h} (w_{hi} - \overline{W}_h)^2,$$

and, from the stratified sampling theory (Sect. 1.2.4),

$$\mathrm{var}[\widehat{\mu}_{HH,st}] = \frac{1}{N^2} \sum_{h=1}^{H} N_h (N_h - n_h) \frac{\sigma_h^2}{n_h}. \tag{4.14}$$

An unbiased estimate of this variance is obtained by replacing σ_h^2 by

$$s_h^2 = \frac{1}{n_h - 1} \sum_{i=1}^{n_h} (w_{hi} - \overline{w}_h)^2.$$

Other unbiased estimates are available including less efficient ones obtained by stopping the adaptive process at the stratum boundary or by not using any units added through crossing stratum boundaries. Here one can use an HT or HH estimator for each stratum and, since the stratum estimates are independent, they can be combined using weights in the usual manner (see Thompson and Seber 1996, Sect. 4.9, and Thompson 1991b). The Rao-Blackwell method can also be applied here.

References

Acharya, B., A. Bhattarai, A. De Gier, and A. Stein. 2000. "Systematic Adaptive Cluster Sampling for the Assessment of Rare Tree Species in Nepal." *Forest Ecology and Management* 137:65–73.

Borkowski, J.J. 1999. "Network Inclusion Probabilities and Horvitz-Thompson Estimation for Adaptive Simple Latin Square Sampling." *Environmental and Ecological Statistics* 6:291–311.

Borkowski, J.J. 2003. "Simple Latin Square Sampling ±k Designs." *Communications in Statistics—Theory and Methods* 32:215–237.

Christman, M.C. 2000. "A Review of Quadrat-Based Sampling of Rare, Geographically Clustered Populations." *Journal of Agricultural, Biological, and Environmental Statistics* 5:168–201.

Félix-Medina, M.H., and S.K. Thompson. 2004. "Adaptive Cluster Double Sampling." *Biometrika* 91:877–891.

Hung, Y. 2011. "Adaptive Probability-Based Latin Hypercube Designs." *Journal of the American Statistical Association, Theory and Methods* 106(493):213–219. DOI: 10.1198/jasa.2011.tm10337.

Munholland, P.L. and J.J. Borkowski. 1993. Adaptive Latin square sampling +1 designs. Technical Report No. 3-23-93, Department of Mathematical Sciences, Montana State University, Bozeman.

Munholland, P.-L., and J.J. Borkowski. 1996. "Latin Square Sampling +1 Designs." *Biometrics* 52:125–136.

Pollard, J.H., D. Palka, and S.T. Buckland. 2002. "Adaptive Line Transect Sampling." *Biometrics* 58(4): 862–870.

Rocco, E. 2008. "Two-Stage Restricted Adaptive Cluster Sampling." *METRON-International Journal of Statistics* LXVI (3):313–327.

Salehi, M.M. 2002. "Systematic Simple Latin Square Sampling (+1) Design and Its Optimality." *Journal of Propagations on Probability and Statistics* 2:191–200.

Salehi, M.M. 2004. "Optimal Sampling Design under a Spatial Correlation Model." *Journal of Statistical Planning and Inference* 118:8–19.

Salehi, M.M. 2006. "Row and Column Elimination Sampling +1 Design." *Communications in Statistics, Theory and Methods* 35(2): 349–362.

Salehi, M.M., and G.A.F. Seber. 1997. "Two-Stage Adaptive Cluster Sampling." *Biometrics* 53:959–970.

Salehi, M.M., and G.A.F. Seber. 2002. "Unbiased Estimators for Restricted Adaptive Cluster Sampling." *Australian and New Zealand Journal of Statistics* 44:63–74.

Särndal, C.E., B. Swensson, and J. Wretman. 1992. *Model Assisted Survey Sampling*. New York: Springer-Verlag.

Thompson, S.K. 1991a. "Adaptive Cluster Sampling: Designs with Primary and Secondary Units." *Biometrics* 47:1103–1115.

Thompson, S.K. 1991b. "Stratified Adaptive Cluster Sampling." *Biometrika* 78:389–397.

Thompson, S.K., and G.A.F. Seber. 1996. *Adaptive Sampling*. New York: Wiley.

Chapter 5
Inverse Sampling Methods

Abstract Inverse sampling is an adaptive method whereby it is the sample size that is adaptive. On the basis of a new proof, Murthy's estimator can now be applied with or without adaptive cluster sampling to inverse sampling to provide unbiased estimators of the mean and variance of the mean estimator. A number of sequential plans along with parameter estimates are considered including a general inverse sampling design, multiple inverse sampling when subpopulation sizes are known, quota sampling, multiple inverse sampling, and truncated multiple inverse sampling.

Keywords Inverse sampling · Murthy's estimator · General inverse sampling design · Quota sampling · Multiple inverse sampling · Truncated multiple inverse sampling

5.1 Introduction

Inverse sampling is an adaptive sampling technique where the sample size is adaptive in that it depends on the incoming information. The technique is credited to Haldane (1945)[1] when he used inverse sampling to estimate the frequency of a rare event. The inclusion probability of a rare event may be so small that, under a fixed-sample size design, not enough cases of interest are selected to estimate either the attribute of interest or to use a statistical method like the contingency table to analysis the data. Inverse sampling can be described generally as a method that requires observations to be continued until certain specified conditions that depend on the results of those observations have been fulfilled. Under this definition many sequential sampling plans can be consider as inverse sampling such as fixed cost sequential sampling (Pathak 1976) and restricted adaptive cluster sampling (Brown and Manly 1998). However, we shall focus on the more traditional inverse sampling where the sampling

---

[1] See Berzofsky, 2008.

G. A. F. Seber and M. M. Salehi, *Adaptive Sampling Designs*, SpringerBriefs in Statistics,   49
DOI: 10.1007/978-3-642-33657-7_5, © The Author(s) 2013

is continued until a predetermined number of individuals have been observed. In Sect. 1.2.3 we introduced Murthy's estimator and we now give a different proof from Salehi and Seber (2001) using the Rao-Blackwell theorem that allows the estimator to be used for more general sampling schemes.

5.2 New Proof of Murthy's Estimator

We begin by assuming that the sample size may be random and we define v to be the number of distinct units in the sample so that $s_R = \{i_1, i_2, \ldots, i_v\}$, the unordered distinct units. Let J_i be an indicator variable that takes the value 1 (with probability p_i) when the ith unit is selected as the first unit, and 0 otherwise. As $E[J_i] = p_i$, a trivial unbiased estimator of μ is given by

$$\widehat{\mu} = \frac{1}{N} \sum_{i=1}^{N} \frac{y_i}{p_i} J_i.$$

Since D_R, the random variable with value $d_R = \{(i, y_i) : i \in s_R\}$ is sufficient for $\theta = (y_1, y_2, \ldots, y_N)'$ (by Theorem 1 in Sect. 3.2), we can use the Rao-Blackwell theorem to obtain the unbiased estimator

$$\widehat{\mu}_{RB} = E[\widehat{\mu} \mid D_R]$$

$$= \frac{1}{N} \sum_{i=1}^{N} \frac{y_i}{p_i} E[J_i \mid D_R]$$

$$= \frac{1}{N} \sum_{i=1}^{N} \frac{y_i}{p_i} \Pr(J_i = 1 \mid D_R)$$

$$= \frac{1}{N} \sum_{i=1}^{N} \frac{y_i}{p_i} \frac{\Pr(J_i = 1, s_R)}{P(s_R)} \tag{5.1}$$

$$= \frac{1}{N} \sum_{i=1}^{v} \frac{P(s_R \mid i)}{P(s_R)} y_i \tag{5.2}$$

$$= \widehat{\mu}_M,$$

as $P(s_R \mid i) = 0$ if the unit i is not in s_R. We see then that $\widehat{\mu}_{RB}$ is Murthy's estimate (Murthy 1957) given in Sect. 1.2.3, and the fraction $P(s_R \mid i)/P(s_R)$ can be evaluated when the associated probabilities are known for the units in s_R, whether or not the sample size v is random. With this new derivation, the estimator $\widehat{\mu}_{RB}$ can now be applied to sequential and adaptive designs as well as to fixed-size sampling designs. Salehi and Seber (2001) showed that the variance formula and its unbiased estimate in Sect. 1.2.3 still hold for these more general sampling schemes.

5.3 Inverse Sampling Design

Following Salehi and Seber (2004), we begin by dividing the population into two subpopulations according to whether or not the units satisfy a certain condition C. A possible condition might be $C = \{y_i > 0\}$ where y_i is the number of individuals in unit i. Denote the two subpopulations by $\mathcal{P}_M$, satisfying the condition and containing M units with population mean μ_M and variance σ_M^2 (with a divisor of $M - 1$), and by $\mathcal{P}_{N-M}$, not satisfying the condition and containing $N - M$ units with population mean μ_{N-M} and variance σ_{N-M}^2 (with a divisor of $N - M - 1$). Suppose we have simple random sampling (i.e., without replacement) and the sampling stops when k units from $\mathcal{P}_M$ are sampled, where k is predetermined. The final sample size, say n_1, will be random. Let $\mathcal{S}_M$ and $\mathcal{S}_{N-M}$ respectively denote the index set of units in the inverse sample that are members of $\mathcal{P}_M$ and $\mathcal{P}_{N-M}$.

To use Eq. (5.1), we need to evaluate the ratio $r = P(s_R \mid i)/P(s_R)$ by determining the number of ordered samples leading to s_R and $\{J_i = 1, s_R\}$. Now let s_C denote those k selected units satisfying C which, for convenience, we index as $i = 1, 2, \ldots, k$. Similarly we let $s_{\bar{C}}$ denote the $n_1 - k$ units that do not satisfy C and index these as $i = k+1, k+2, \ldots, n_1$. Since the last observation must satisfy C, we see that after allocating one of the k sample units satisfying C the rest can be ordered in $(n_1 - 1)!$ ways. The sample s_R can therefore be constructed in $k \times (n_1 - 1)!$ ways. For the unit i in the set s_C the event $\{J_i = 1, s_R\}$ can occur in $(k - 1) \times (n_1 - 2)!$ ways, while if it is in the set $s_{\bar{C}}$ it can occur in $k \times (n_1 - 2)!$ ways. Since $p_i = 1/N$ for all i, the ratio r will have only two values so that from (5.1) with $v = n_1$ we get a weighted sample mean

$$
\begin{aligned}
\widehat{\mu}_{RB} &= \sum_{i=1}^{k} y_i \frac{(k - 1) \times (n_1 - 2)!}{k \times (n_1 - 1)!} + \sum_{i=k+1}^{n_1} y_i \frac{k \times (n_1 - 2)!}{k \times (n_1 - 1)!} \\
&= \widehat{P}\overline{y}_M + (1 - \widehat{P})\overline{y}_{N-M},
\end{aligned}
\tag{5.3}
$$

where

$$
\widehat{P} = \frac{k - 1}{n_1 - 1}, \quad \overline{y}_M = \frac{1}{k} \sum_{i \in \mathcal{S}_M} y_i, \text{ and } \overline{y}_{N-M} = \frac{1}{n_1 - k} \sum_{i \in \mathcal{S}_{N-M}} y_i.
$$

It turns out, as we shall see below, that $\widehat{P}$ is an unbiased estimator of M/N. To find an unbiased estimator of the variance of $\widehat{\mu}_{RB}$, we can use the formulas in Sect. 1.2.3. We need to compute $P(s_R \mid i, j)$, the probability that units i and j are the first two selected units. Arguing as above, we find that for $k > 2$,

$$\frac{P(s_R \mid i, j)}{P(s_R)} = \begin{cases} \dfrac{N(N-1)(k-2)}{(n_1-1)(n_1-2)k}, & \text{if } i, j \in s_C, \\[3mm] \dfrac{N(N-1)(k-1)}{(n_1-1)(n_1-2)k}, & \text{if } i \in s_C \text{ and } j \in s_{\bar{C}}, \\[3mm] \dfrac{N(N-1)}{(n_1-1)(n_1-2)}, & \text{if } i \in s_{\bar{C}}. \end{cases}$$

Substituting for the various probabilities, we have from Sect. 1.2.3 the following unbiased variance estimator, namely (Salehi and Seber 2004)

$$\widehat{\text{var}}[\widehat{\mu}_{RB}] = \sum_{i=1}^{n_1} \sum_{j<i}^{n_1} \left(\frac{P(s_R \mid i, j)}{P(s_R)} - \frac{P(s_R \mid i)P(s_R \mid j)}{[P(s_R)]^2} \right) \left(\frac{y_i}{Np_i} - \frac{y_j}{Np_j} \right)^2 p_i p_j$$

$$= \frac{1}{N(n_1-1)^2(n_1-2)} \left\{ c \sum_{i=1}^{k} \sum_{j<i}^{k} (y_i - y_j)^2 \right.$$

$$\left. + \frac{N - n_1 + 1}{N^2} \left(\frac{k-1}{k} \sum_{i=1}^{k} \sum_{j=k+1}^{n_1} (y_i - y_j)^2 + \sum_{i=k+1}^{n_1} \sum_{j>i}^{n_1} (y_i - y_j)^2 \right) \right\}$$

$$= \widehat{P}^2 \left(\frac{(N - n_1 + 1)(n_1 k - n_1 - k) - N(n_1 - 2)}{N(n_1 - 2)(k - 1)} \right) \frac{s_M^2}{k}$$

$$+ \widehat{\text{var}}[\widehat{P}](\bar{y}_M - \bar{y}_{N-M})^2 + \left(\frac{(N - n_1 + 1)(n_1 - k - 1)}{N(n_1 - 1)(n_1 - 2)} \right) s_{N-M}^2,$$

$$= a s_M^2 + \widehat{\text{var}}[\widehat{P}](\bar{y}_M - \bar{y}_{N-M})^2 + b s_{N-M}^2, \tag{5.4}$$

where

$$c = \frac{k(k-2)(N - n_1 + 1) - N(n_1 - 2)}{k^2},$$

$$a = \frac{\widehat{P}^2(N - n_1 + 1)(n_1 k - n_1 - k) - N(n_1 - 2)}{N(n_1 - 2)k(k - 1)},$$

$$b = \frac{(N - n_1 + 1)(n_1 - k - 1)}{N(n_1 - 1)(n_1 - 2)} \tag{5.5}$$

$$\widehat{\text{var}}[\widehat{P}] = \frac{(n_1 - k)(k - 1)(N - n_1 + 1)}{N(n_1 - 1)^2(n_1 - 2)} = \left(1 - \frac{n_1 - 1}{N} \right) \frac{\widehat{P}(N - \widehat{P})}{n_1 - 2},$$

$$s_M^2 = \frac{1}{k-1} \sum_{i=1}^{k} (y_i - \bar{y}_M)^2, \quad \text{and} \quad s_{N-M}^2 = \frac{1}{n_1 - k - 1} \sum_{i=k+1}^{n_1} (y_i - \bar{y}_{N-M})^2.$$

The above formulas can also be derived using properties of the hypergeometric distribution, as in Greco and Naddeo (2007). They also derived formulas for inverse sampling with replacement.

In some situations we are particularly interested in the ratio $P = M/N$, the number of units with a particular characteristic. This is the same as estimating μ when y_i is an indicator variable taking the value 1 if the unit possesses the desired characteristic and zero otherwise. From (5.1) we have the estimator

$$\widehat{P} = \frac{k-1}{n_1 - 1}.$$

Since $n_1 p_i = 1$, the second equation of (5.4) contains terms of the form $y_i - y_j$ that will be zero when y_i and y_j are both 1, or equal to one if just one is zero. We therefore need to evaluate only $\sum_{i=1}^{k} \sum_{j=k+1}^{n_1} (y_i - y_j)^2 = k(n_1 - k)$ and then substitute into the second equation of (5.4) to get the unbiased variance estimate (Salehi and Seber 2001, p. 284)

$$\widehat{\text{var}}[\widehat{P}] = \frac{(n_1 - k)(k-1)(N - n_1 + 1)}{N(n_1 - 1)^2(n_1 - 2)} = \left(1 - \frac{n_1 - 1}{N}\right) \frac{\widehat{P}(1 - \widehat{P})}{n_1 - 1}.$$

A special case of this is when the unit contains only one object so that P is the population proportion of objects with a certain characteristic (e.g., left-handedness). The above theory can be readily modified to take care of the case when sampling is with replacement (See Salehi and Seber 2001, p. 284).

Aggarwal and Pandey (2010) have used inverse sampling to estimate the prevalence of the disease burden due to leprosy in an endemic area of Uttar Pradesh, India. They concluded that inverse sampling was found to be feasible as compared to conventional sampling in terms of less time consumed, low cost, and less population covered. They believed that the method could be adopted at a national level.

Greco and Naddeo (2007) derived an unbiased estimator of the population total as well as unbiased estimators of the two subpopulations totals, their variances, and the corresponding variance estimators in inverse sampling with replacement when the units have unequal selection probabilities.

In some situations we may know the size of subpopulations (Chang et al. 1998). Mohammadi and Salehi (2011) derived the Horvitz-Thompson estimator for the population mean under inverse sampling designs when the sizes of subpopulations are known. They also considered another unbiased weighted estimator based on post-stratification. They compared the precisions of the proposed estimators and found that they depend on the coefficient of variation of two subpopulations and the square of the less-interesting subpopulation mean. The Horvitz-Thompson estimator is sensitive to distance of the subpopulation mean from zero, while the alternative estimator is more stable.

5.4 General Inverse Sampling Design

Christman and Lan (2001) considered the following three inverse sampling designs that use stopping rules based on the number of rare units observed in the sample:

(i) We select units one at a time until we have obtained a predetermined number of rare units, say k, in the sample, which is "ordinary" inverse sampling.

(ii) We first select an initial simple random sample of size n_0. If the number of rare units is greater than or equal to k we stop sampling, otherwise we keep sampling until we observe k rare units.

(iii) This is similar to design (ii) but with the difference that we stop sampling if the initial sample of size n_0 contains at least one rare unit. Otherwise, we keep sampling until we observe k rare units.

The authors presented unbiased estimators and some intermediate expressions for their variances for designs (i) and (ii). They also presented a biased estimator for design (iii). Appropriate variance estimators were not provided, apart from some bounds based on Mikulski and Smith (1976).

Salehi and Seber (2004) derived an unbiased estimator for the sampling design (iii) as well as unbiased variance estimators for the three sampling designs using Murthy's formula. They introduced a more practical sampling design which is essentially sampling design (ii), but with sampling stopping when one runs out of resources (e.g., money or time). They called it the General Inverse Sampling (GIS) design as simple random sampling and sampling designs (i) and (ii) are special cases of it. This design begins with a simple random sample of size n_0 with sampling stopping if at least k units from $\mathcal{P}_M$ are selected. Otherwise, we sequentially continue sampling until either exactly k units from $\mathcal{P}_M$ are selected or n_2 units are selected in total. This sampling design is design (ii), but a limit is put on final sample size; design (ii) corresponds to $n_2 = N$. If $n_2 = n_1$, general inverse sampling reduces to simple random sampling, while if $n_0 = 1$ and $n_2 = N$ we have design (i).

We now apply Murthy's estimator to the GIS design to get

$$
\widehat{\mu}_{GIS} = \begin{cases} \dfrac{1}{n_0} \displaystyle\sum_{i=1}^{n_0} y_i, & \text{if } [Q_1], \\[2ex] \hat{P}\bar{y}_M + (1 - \hat{P})\bar{y}_{N-M}, & \text{if } [Q_2], \\[2ex] \dfrac{1}{n_2} \displaystyle\sum_{i=1}^{n_2} y_i, & \text{if } [Q_3], \end{cases} \tag{5.6}
$$

where $[Q_1] = \{n_1 = n_0\}$, $[Q_2] = \{n_0 < n_1 < n_2\}$ or $\{n_1 = n_2$ and $|\mathcal{S}_M| = k\}$, $[Q_3] = \{n_1 = n_2$ and $|\mathcal{S}_M| < k\}$, and $|\mathcal{S}_M|$ is the cardinality (size) of $\mathcal{S}_M$. An unbiased estimator of $\text{var}[\widehat{\mu}_{GIS}]$ is

$$\widehat{var}[\hat{\mu}_{GIS}] = \begin{cases} \left(1 - \dfrac{n_0}{N}\right) \dfrac{s_0^2}{n_0}, & \text{if } [Q_1], \\[2mm] as_M^2 + \widehat{var}[\widehat{P}](\bar{y}_M - \bar{y}_{N-M})^2 + bs_{N-M}^2, & \text{if } [Q_2], \\[2mm] \left(1 - \dfrac{n_2}{N}\right) \dfrac{s_2^2}{n_2}, & \text{if } [Q_3], \end{cases} \tag{5.7}$$

where a and b are given by (5.5), $s_r^2 = (n_r - 1)^{-1} \sum_{i=1}^{n_r}(y_i - \bar{y}_r)^2$ and $\bar{y}_r = (n_r)^{-1} \sum_{i=1}^{n_r} y_i$ (for $r = 0, 2$).

Salehi and Seber (2004) also incorporated adaptive cluster sampling with general inverse sampling designs for the case when the rare events tend to be clumped—the typical sparse but clustered population.

Moradi et al. (2007) considered the problem of estimating a ratio for which the denominator of the estimator can take a zero value. Under a simple random sampling (SRS) design, if all observations of the denominator variable are zero, the ratio estimator would be undefined. A natural solution is to use an inverse sampling design for which one continues sampling until at least a predetermined number of nonzero values is observed for the denominator variable. Using Taylor linearization, they derived an asymptotic unbiased estimator of the ratio and an approximate variance estimator of its variance for a general inverse sampling design.

Their simulation study was based on a survey of honey production in the Kurdistan Province of Iran conducted by the Statistical Center of Iran (SCI). On the basis of a request from an organization, the SCI enumerated all cities and villages with the aim of measuring the total amount of honey produced, as well as the amount of honey produced per family in Kurdistan. The major objective of this census was to construct a sampling frame for an annual sample survey which will be performed by that organization. Families in villages of Kurdistan live together in a relatively small region and they know what other people do in their home village. It is not difficult to find out which families have honey farms by asking an adult in the village. Also, there are some organizations in the cities that know honey farm owners. Therefore, a preliminary proposal was to consider cities and villages as sampling units and to use a simple random sampling of cities and villages. If, however, we were to use simple random sampling, it would be likely that none of the families sampled in the selected villages has a honey farm since the number of such farms is not large. In this instance, the estimator of the ratio would be undefined. If we were to use inverse sampling, its ratio estimator would always be well-defined, but, the lack of a predefined fixed sample size would make it difficult to plan budgets and survey logistics. However, use of a general inverse sampling approach would avoid the scenario of an undefined estimator and allow us to plan the costs and operations of the survey.

Moradi et al. (2011) introduced regression estimators for the general inverse sampling design and inverse sampling with unequal selection probabilities. For both, the variances of regression estimators as well as variance estimators were developed. Using a simulation study on a real population, that is, arsenic contamination in a region of Kurdistan, they showed that regression estimators are more efficient than their counterparts. In inverse sampling with unequal selection probabilities, arsenic concentration in the plant was the y-value (or response variable in a regression context), the arsenic concentration in the water (z_i) was used to compute the probability of selection p_i ($= z_i / \sum z_j$), and the arsenic concentration in the soil was considered as an auxiliary sampling variable (the explanatory variable in a regression model).

5.5 Multiple Inverse Sampling

Chang et al. (1998) introduced a sequential sampling procedure named Multiple Inverse Sampling (MIS) and supposed that the population can be partitioned into subpopulations with known sizes. They employed the MIS to avoid the undesirable events of obtaining no sample unit or a very small number of sampled units from some post-strata in a post-stratified sampling design. Through simulation they found the MIS reasonably efficient. There are many situations where we don't know the subpopulation that a unit belongs to until the unit is sampled, nor know the subpopulation sizes. There are also situations where one of the objectives of a sample survey is to estimate subpopulation sizes, for example, the estimation of animal numbers in different age categories, and the estimation of household frequencies using different heating or cooling systems in energy consumption surveys.

Salehi and Chang (2005) extended the use of Murthy's estimator from the traditional inverse sampling to the multiple case. They developed unbiased estimators (and their unbiased variance estimators) of τ, the total population y-value, as well as the y-totals for subpopulations using Murthy's estimator. They also incorporated the sampling design in Chang et al. (1998) of starting with a simple random sample but truncating the sampling at some stage (Chang et al. 1999).

5.5.1 Quota Sampling

Quota sampling (see Scheaffer et al. 1990, p. 25) can be a version of the MIS design in the finite population context. In fact quota sampling is somewhat notorious as it has been misused by some inexperienced practitioners. The MIS improves quota sampling in the sense that it provides some theoretical basis, including a properly designed stopping rule followed by a well-developed estimation methodology, as opposed to the misuse of human subjectivity in quota sampling. In this sampling design, researchers first select a simple random sample from the whole population. If it happens that some of the subpopulations are under-represented in the sample set, the researchers would select more units one at a time until the sample sizes of those under-represented subpopulations reach some satisfactory level. Practitioners usually use quota sampling and then suppose that the sample was selected at random using simple random sampling estimators, which are biased. For example, Sarraf-Zadegan et al. (2003) used a similar sampling procedure in a study on cardiovascular disease. They partitioned Isfahan into 93 Primary Sample Units (PSUs). Each PSU had approximately 1000 households, and they randomly selected 25 PSUs. Approximately 5–10 percent of households within those selected PSUs were selected. One individual with age over 19 years per household was randomly selected if mentally competent, and not pregnant if a woman. In practice, whenever the sample sizes from some of age subpopulations (19–24, 25–34, 35–44, 45–54, 55–64 and $\geq$65) were smaller than predetermined values (which were set to match the community age distribution), more households were randomly selected. This was done one household at a time, and one individual aged over 19 years was randomly selected from each selected household until the sample sizes of all age subpopulations were as large as the predetermined values. They referred to their sampling design as quota sampling. If the desired sample sizes in each subpopulation are set before the field work, then quota sampling is actually the MIS design.

The properties of the introduced sampling designs and their estimators of the total y-values of subpopulations depend on the distribution of the variable of interest. In order to evaluate the introduced sampling design and their estimators regardless of the distribution of the variable of interest, Salehi and Chang (2005) developed estimators and their variance estimators for the proportions (weights) of subpopulations when the sampling design is Truncated Multiple Inverse Sampling (Chang et al. 1999). Using a simulation study, it was found that for this sampling design the estimators are reasonably efficient for estimating the proportions of rare subpopulations. We now give some theory for this method.

5.5.2 Truncated Multiple Inverse Sampling

Suppose that population $\mathcal{P} = \{u_1, u_2, \ldots, u_N\}$, where u_i is the ith unit, can be divided into L subpopulations $\mathcal{P}_h$ ($h = 1, \ldots, L$). Sampling is without replacement and it is desired that the sample size n_h from subpopulation h be greater than or equal to a predetermined number m_h for all h. Beginning with a simple random sample of size n_0, one sequentially continues sampling until either at least m_h sample units are selected from subpopulation h, for all $h = 1, \ldots, L$, or until n_T units are selected in total. The sample set is partitioned into a set of sampled units for which $n_h = m_h$, say $\mathcal{S}_M$, and a set of sampled units for which $n_h > m_h$, say $\mathcal{S}_{\overline{M}}$. Let $\widehat{p} = (k-1)/(n-1)$, where k is the cardinality of the sample set $\mathcal{S}_M$ and $n = \sum_h n_h$. Using Murthy's estimator, we have from Salehi and Chang (2005, with corrections to the Q_i), the following unbiased estimator of the population mean:

$$
\hat{\mu} =
\begin{cases}
\displaystyle\sum_{h=1}^{L} \frac{n_h}{n_0} \bar{y}_h, & \text{if } [Q_1], \\[2ex]
\displaystyle\sum_{h \in \mathcal{S}_M} \frac{n_h \hat{p}}{k} \bar{y}_h + \sum_{h \in \mathcal{S}_{\bar{M}}} \frac{n_h(1-\hat{p})}{n-k} \bar{y}_h, & \text{if } [Q_2], \\[2ex]
\displaystyle\sum_{h=1}^{L} \frac{n_h}{n_T} \bar{y}_h, & \text{if } [Q_3],
\end{cases}
$$

where $[Q_1] = \{n = n_0\}$, $[Q_2] = \{n_0 < n < n_T\}$ or $\{n = n_T$ and $n_h \geq m_h$ for all $h\}$, and $[Q_3] = \{n = n_T$ and $n_h < m_h$ for at least one $h\}$. Its variance estimator is given by

$$
\widehat{\mathrm{var}}[\hat{\mu}] =
\begin{cases}
\left(1 - \dfrac{n_0}{N}\right)\dfrac{s_0^2}{n_0}, & \text{if } [Q_1], \\[3ex]
\hat{p}^2\left(\dfrac{(N-n+1)(nk-n-k) - N(n-2)}{N(n-2)(k-1)}\right)\dfrac{s_M^2}{k} & \text{if } [Q_2] \\[3ex]
\quad + \widehat{\mathrm{var}}[\hat{p}](\bar{y}_M - \bar{y}_{\bar{M}})^2 + \left(\dfrac{(N-n+1)(n-k-1)}{N(n-1)(n-2)}\right)s_{\bar{M}}^2, & \\[3ex]
\left(1 - \dfrac{n_T}{N}\right)\dfrac{s_1^2}{n_T}, & \text{if } [Q_3],
\end{cases}
$$

where $s_1^2 = (n_T - 1)^{-1}\sum_{i=1}^{n_T}(y_i - \bar{y}_1)^2$, $\bar{y}_1 = n_T^{-1}\sum_{i=1}^{n_T} y_i$, $\bar{y}_M = (1/k)\sum_{i \in \mathcal{S}_M} y_i$ and $\bar{y}_{\bar{M}} = [1/(n-k)]\sum_{i \in \mathcal{S}_{\bar{M}}} y_i$. An estimator of the mean for subpopulation h, say $\hat{\mu}_h$, is

$$
\hat{\mu}_h =
\begin{cases}
\dfrac{n_h}{n_0} \bar{y}_h, & \text{if } [Q_1], \\[2ex]
\dfrac{n_h \hat{p}}{k} \bar{y}_h, & \text{if } [Q_2] \text{ and } \mathbf{S}_h \subseteq \mathcal{S}_M, \\[2ex]
\dfrac{n_h(1-\hat{p})}{n-k} \bar{y}_h & \text{if } [Q_2] \text{ and } \mathbf{S}_h \subseteq \mathcal{S}_{\bar{M}}, \\[2ex]
\dfrac{n_h}{n_T} \bar{y}_h, & \text{if } [Q_3],
\end{cases}
$$

where $\mathbf{S}_h$ is the sample set from subpopulation h. Its variance estimator is

$$\widehat{\mathrm{var}}[\hat{\mu}_h] = \begin{cases} (1 - \dfrac{n_0}{N})\dfrac{s_0^{*2}}{n_0}, & \text{if } [Q_1], \\[2ex] \hat{p}^2 \left(\dfrac{(N-n+1)(nk-n-k)-N(n-2)}{N(n-2)(k-1)} \right) \dfrac{s_M^{*2}}{k} & \text{if } [Q_2] \text{ and } \mathbf{S}_h \subseteq \mathcal{S}_M, \\ \quad + N^2 \widehat{\mathrm{var}}[\hat{p}]\, \bar{y}_M^{*2}, \\[2ex] \left(\dfrac{(N-n+1)(n-k-1)}{N(n-1)(n-2)} \right) s_{\bar{M}}^{*2} & \text{if } [Q_2] \text{ and } \mathbf{S}_h \subseteq \mathcal{S}_{\bar{M}}, \\ \quad + \widehat{\mathrm{var}}[\hat{p}]\, \bar{y}_{\bar{M}}^{*2}, \\[2ex] (1 - \dfrac{n_T}{N})\dfrac{s_1^{*2}}{n_T}, & \text{if } [Q_3], \end{cases}$$

where s_0^{*2}, s_1^{*2}, $\bar{y}_M^{*2}$ and $\bar{y}_{\bar{M}}^{*2}$ are respectively s_0^2, s_1^2, $\bar{y}_M^2$ and $\bar{y}_{\bar{M}}^2$, evaluated for the following variable

$$y_i^* = \begin{cases} y_i & \text{if } i \text{ is in subpopulation h} \\ 0 & \text{if } i \text{ is not in subpopulation h.} \end{cases}$$

Multiple inverse sampling is an appropriate sampling design for collecting data for categorical data analysis. Salehi et al. (2006) extended the methods for using multiple logistic regression to sample surveys that have MIS designs.

References

Aggarwal, A., A. Pandey. 2010. "Inverse Sampling to Study Disease Burden of Leprosy". *The Indian Journal of Medical Research* 132:438–441.

Berzofsky, M. 2008. "Inverse Sampling". In P.J. Lavrakas (Ed.), *Encyclopedia of Survey Research Methods*. Thousand Oaks, CA: Sage Publications.

Brown, J., and B.F.J. Manly. 1998. "Restricted Adaptive Cluster Sampling". *Journal of Ecological and Environmental Statistics* 5(1):47–62.

Chang, K-C., J.F. Liu, and C.P. Han. 1998. "Multiple Inverse Sampling in Post-Stratification". *Journal of Statistical Planning and Inference* 69: 209–227.

Chang, K-C., C.P. Han, and D.L. Hawkins. 1999. "Truncated Multiple Inverse Sampling in Post-Stratification". *Journal of Statistical Planning and Inference* 76:215–234.

Christman, M.C., and F. Lan. 2001. "Inverse Adaptive Cluster Sampling". *Biometrics* 57:1096–1105.

Greco L., and S. Naddeo. 2007. "Inverse Sampling with Unequal Selection Probabilities". *Communications in Statistics—Theory and Methods* 36(5):1039–1048.

Haldane, J.B.S. (1945). "On a Method of Estimating Frequencies". *Biometrika* 33:222–225.

Mikulski, P. W., and P.J. Smith. 1976. "A Variance Bound for Unbiased Estimation in Inverse Sampling". *Biometrika* 63:216–217.

Mohammadi, M., and M.M. Salehi. 2011. "Horvitz Thompson Estimator of Population Mean Under Inverse Sampling Designs". *Bulletin of the Iranian Mathematical Society*. In press.

Moradi, M., M.M. Salehi, and P.S. Levy. 2007. "Using General Inverse Sampling Design to Avoid Undefined Estimator". *Journal of Probability and Statistical Science* 5(2):137–150.

Moradi M., M. Salehi, J.A. Brown, and N. Karimie. 2011."Regression Estimator Under Inverse Sampling to Estimate Arsenic Contamination". *Environmetrics*, DOI: 10.1002/env.1116.

Murthy, M.N. 1957. "Ordered and Unordered Estimators in Sampling without Replacement". *Sankhyā* 18:379–390.

Pathak, P.K. 1976. "Unbiased Estimation in Fixed Cost Sequential Sampling Schemes". *The Annals of Statistics* 4:1012–1017.

Salehi M.M., and G.A.F. Seber. 2001. "A New Proof of Murthy's Estimator Which Applies to Sequential Sampling". *Australian and New Zealand Journal of Statistics* 43(3):901–906.

Salehi, M.M., and G.A.F. Seber. 2004. "A General Inverse Sampling Scheme and Its Application to Adaptive Cluster Sampling". *Australian and New Zealand Journal of Statistics* 46:483–494.

Salehi M.M., and K-C. Chang 2005. "Multiple Inverse Sampling in Post-stratification with Sub-population Sizes Unknown: A Solution for Quota Sampling". *Journal of Statistical Planning and Inference* 131(2):379–392.

Salehi, M.M., P.S. Levy, M.A. Jamalzadeh, and Chang, K.-C. 2006."Adaptation of Multiple Logistic Regression to a Multiple Inverse Sampling Design: Application to the Isfahan Healthy Heart Program". *Statistics in Medicine* 25:1 71–85.

Sarraf-Zadegan, N., Gh. Sadri, H.A. Malek, M. Baghaei, F.N. Mohammadi, and others. 2003. "Isfahan Healthy Heart Programme: a Comprehensive Integrated Community-Based Programme for Cardiovascular Disease Prevention and Control. Design, Methods and Initial Experience". *Acta Cardiologica* 58:309–320.

Scheaffer, R.L., W. Mendenhall, and L. Ott. 1990. *Elementary Survey Sampling*, 4th edit. Boston: PWS-KENT.

Chapter 6
Adaptive Allocation

Abstract Adaptive allocation is a form of sampling whereby information from an initial phase of sampling is use to allocate the effort for further sampling, usually referred to as the the second phase. The material in this chapter is an extension of the material of the previous chapter with its emphasis on stratified sampling and two-stage sampling. A number of allocation schemes from several authors including those of Francis, Jolly and Hampton, Salehi and Smith, Brown et al., Salehi et al., and Salehi and Brown are described.

Keywords Adaptive allocation · Stratified sampling · Two-phase designs

6.1 Introduction

In conventional stratified sampling, the population is divided into regions or strata and a simple random sample is taken from each stratum, with the sample selection in one stratum being independent of selections in the others. We wish to obtain the best estimate of τ, the population total of y-values, subject to having a prescribed total sample size or total survey cost, or else achieving a desired precision with minimum cost. It transpires that the optimal allocation of the total sample among the strata results in larger sample sizes in strata that are larger, more variable, and less costly to sample (Cochran 1977; Thompson and Seber 1996).

If prior knowledge of the strata variances is not available, it would be natural to carry out the sampling in two phases and compute either sample variances or use measurements representing the variances from the first phase. These are then used to adaptively allocate the reminder of the sampling effort among the strata. This allocation could be based on the stratum sample mean or on the number of large values in the first phase sample rather than sample variances, since with many natural populations high means or large values are associated with high variances. As we saw in Sect. 1.2.4, the standard stratified sampling estimator gives an unbiased estimator of the population total with conventional stratified random sampling but it is not in general unbiased with adaptive allocation designs.

G. A. F. Seber and M. M. Salehi, *Adaptive Sampling Designs*, SpringerBriefs in Statistics, DOI: 10.1007/978-3-642-33657-7_6, © The Author(s) 2013

In this chapter, we first present the basic theory. We then review some recently developed adaptive allocation sampling designs. We may classify such a design as either having a variable sample size or fixed sample size. The former has the advantage that the allocation of the second-phase effort can also be done during the first phase, which means that the stratum that is to be surveyed in the second phase will not need to be revisited; such a revisit may be costly. However, it has the disadvantage of having an unknown final sample size prior to surveying. This can make planning the survey difficult. On the other hand, one knows the size of the final sample for a fixed sample-size design, but some strata may have to be revisited.

6.2 Basic Theory

6.2.1 Initial Simple Random Samples

Suppose we have H strata with n_h units in stratum h ($h = 1, 2, \ldots, H$) so that the total number of units is $N = \sum_{h=1}^{H} N_h$. Let y_{hj} be the y-value for the jth unit in stratum h. In the first phase we take a simple random sample (without replacement) of size n_{h1} from stratum h for each stratum. If a certain criterion C such as $\overline{y}_{h1} > c$ is satisfied, where $\overline{y}_{h1}$ is the sample mean for the units sampled in stratum h, we take a second sample of size n_{h2} from that stratum. Our first step is to find an unbiased estimate of the mean μ_h and of its associated variance estimate. Any pair will do to use the Rao-Blackwell modification for stratum h, so we can use the data from just phase 1 to begin with. This leads to unbiased estimates $\overline{y}_{h1}$ and s_{h1}^2 of μ_h and σ_h^2, respectively, where

$$\sigma_h^2 = \frac{1}{N_h - 1} \sum_{j=1}^{N_h} (y_{hj} - \mu_h)^2 \quad and \quad s_{h1}^2 = \frac{1}{n_{h1} - 1} \sum_{j=1}^{n_{h1}} (y_{hj} - \overline{y}_{h1}^2)^2. \tag{6.1}$$

Since the unit labels are not used for estimation within strata, we have from Theorem 6 in Sect. 3.4 that $\mathbf{y}_{hR}$, the set of y-values corresponding to the unordered units for the *total* sample (phases 1 and 2) in stratum h, is equivalent to $\mathbf{y}_{h,rank}$ and is therefore a complete sufficient statistic for μ_h. This is good news as, when $n_{h2} > 0$, we can now use the Rao-Blackwell theorem to obtain minimum variance unbiased estimates of μ_h and σ_h^2, namely $\widehat{\mu}_{hRB} = E[\overline{y}_{h1} \mid \mathbf{y}_{hR}]$ and $s_{hRB}^2 = E[s_{h1}^2 \mid \mathbf{y}_{hR}]$.

We now focus on stratum h (with $n_{h2} > 0$) and, to simplify the notation, we drop the suffix h. If $n = n_1 + n_2$ is the total number of observations, we can compute the mean $\overline{y}_{1g}$ of the first n_1 observations using permutation g ($g = 1, 2, \ldots, G$), where $G = n!$ is the number of possible permutations of $\mathbf{y}_R$. Let J_g be an indicator variable taking the value of 1 when condition C is satisfied, and 0 otherwise. Since all G permutations are equally likely, we see that the $\xi = \sum_{g=1}^{G} J_g$ permutations satisfying C are also equally likely and

$$\hat{\mu}_{RB} = E[\bar{y}_1 \mid \mathbf{y}_R]$$

$$= \begin{cases} \dfrac{1}{\xi} \displaystyle\sum_{g=1}^{G} \bar{y}_{1g} J_g, & \xi > 1, \\[2mm] \bar{y}_1, & \xi = 1. \end{cases} \tag{6.2}$$

To find an unbiased estimator of $\mathrm{var}[\hat{\mu}_{RB}]$ we see that (6.2) takes the same form as (3.2) so that the theory of Sect. 3.3 can be applied here. From Eq. (3.1),

$$\mathrm{var}[\hat{\mu}_{RB}] = \mathrm{var}[\bar{y}_1] - E\{\mathrm{var}[\bar{y}_1 \mid \mathbf{y}_R]\},$$

and an unbiased estimator of $\mathrm{var}[\bar{y}_1]$ is $s_1^2(N - n_1)/n_1 N$ (from Sect. 1.2.2). Hence an unbiased estimator of $\mathrm{var}[\hat{\mu}_{RB}]$ is

$$\widehat{\mathrm{var}}[\hat{\mu}_{RB}] = E\{\widehat{\mathrm{var}}[\bar{y}_1]\mid \mathbf{y}_R\} - \mathrm{var}[\bar{y}_1 \mid \mathbf{y}_R]$$

$$= E[s_1^2 \mid \mathbf{y}_R]\left(\frac{1}{n_1} - \frac{1}{N}\right) - \mathrm{var}[\bar{y}_1 \mid \mathbf{y}_R]$$

$$= \begin{cases} \dfrac{1}{\xi} \displaystyle\sum_{g=1}^{\xi} \left\{ s_{1g}^2 \left(\frac{1}{n_1} - \frac{1}{N}\right) - (\bar{y}_{1g} - \hat{\mu}_{RB})^2 \right\}, & \xi > 1, \\[4mm] s_1^2 \left(\dfrac{1}{n_1} - \dfrac{1}{N}\right), & \xi = 1, \end{cases} \tag{6.3}$$

where s_{1g}^2 is the value of s_1^2 calculated from the first n_1 observations using permutation g. The estimators (6.2) and (6.3) were obtained by Kremers (1987). Some simplification of the calculations is possible (Thompson and Seber 1996, p.186). The final step is to combine the stratum estimates in the form (see Sect. 1.2.4)

$$\hat{\mu}_{RB} = \sum_{h=1}^{H} \frac{N_h}{N} \hat{\mu}_{hRB} \quad \text{and} \quad \widehat{\mathrm{var}}[\hat{\mu}_{RB}] = \sum_{h=1}^{H} \frac{N_h^2}{N^2} \widehat{\mathrm{var}}[\hat{\mu}_{hRB}],$$

using (6.2) and (6.3) for each stratum to give unbiased estimators. We note that the rule of sampling further if condition C holds makes good sense in fisheries where the stratum variances tend to increase with stratum means. We take further samples in the strata with greater variability.

6.2.2 Using Observations from Previously Located Strata

We begin with a simple example from shrimp fishing. Suppose the survey area is a bay divided into a grid of strata. Within each stratum a tow is located at random. If more than 50lbs of shrimp per mile are caught, a full mile-tow is made in the next stratum, otherwise a short tow of 1/2 mile is made. The process begins with a 1-mile tow. We now develop the theory for a more general scheme from Thompson et al. (1992).

We use a similar notation to that above, but we shall concentrate on population density $D = \tau/A$, where A is the population area. The study region is partitioned into H strata of area A_h ($h = 1, 2, \ldots, H$), and there are N_h units each of area a_h in stratum h so that $A_h = N_h a_h$. Let τ_h be the sum of the y-values in stratum h and let $\mu_h = \tau_h/N_h$. A simple random sample of n_h units is taken from stratum h and y_{hi} ($h = 1, 2, \ldots, n_h$) is the associated y-value (e.g., number of animals or biomass) in unit i in the sample. Let $\overline{y}_h = \sum_{i=1}^{n_h} y_{hi}$ be the sample mean for stratum h. The stratum density $D_h = \tau_h/A_h$ ($= \mu_h/a_h$) can be estimated by the sample estimate $\widehat{D}_h = \overline{y}_h/a_h$.

The sampling design is as follows. We take a simple random sample of n_1 units from the first stratum. We then take a simple random sample of n_2 units from the second stratum depending on $\widehat{D}_1$. We continue in this fashion selecting n_h units from stratum h with n_h depending on the observed density $\widehat{D}_{h-1}$ in the preceding stratum. The appropriate stratified estimate of D is then

$$\widehat{D} = \sum_{h=1}^{H} W_h \widehat{D}_h, \quad \text{where} \quad W_h = \frac{A_h}{A}. \tag{6.4}$$

If c_h denotes "the set of all $\widehat{D}_k$ for $k < h$", then, since c_h determines n_h, we have that

$$E[\widehat{D}_h \mid c_h] = \frac{1}{a_h} E[\overline{y}_h \mid n_h] = \frac{\mu_h}{a_h} = D_h \quad \text{and} \quad E[\widehat{D}_h] = D_h. \tag{6.5}$$

This implies that

$$E[\widehat{D}] = \sum_h W_h E[\widehat{D}_h] = \sum_h W_h D_h = \sum_h \frac{A_h}{A} D_h = \frac{\tau}{A} = D. \tag{6.6}$$

We also have the following well-known result involving conditional means and variances, namely

$$\text{var}[\widehat{D}_h] = E_{c_h}[\text{var}(\widehat{D}_h \mid c_h)] + \text{var}_{c_h}[E(\widehat{D}_h \mid c_h)] = E_{c_h}[\text{var}(\widehat{D}_h \mid c_h)] \tag{6.7}$$

with the second term being zero by (6.5). Now for $h < i$, c_i will determine $\widehat{D}_h$ so that by (6.5)

$$E[(\widehat{D}_h - D_h)(\widehat{D}_i - D_i) \mid c_i] = (\widehat{D}_h - D_h) E[(\widehat{D}_i - D_i) \mid c_i] = 0.$$

Taking expectations with respect to c_i gives us

$$E[(\widehat{D}_h - D_h)(\widehat{D}_i - D_i)] = 0. \tag{6.8}$$

Applying (6.6) and (6.8)

$$
\begin{aligned}
\text{var}[\widehat{D}] &= \text{E}\left\{\left[\sum_{h=1}^{H} W_h(\widehat{D}_h - D)\right]^2\right\} \\
&= \text{E}\left\{\left[\sum_{h=1}^{H} W_h(\widehat{D}_h - D_h)\right]^2\right\} \\
&= \text{E}\left[\sum_{h=1}^{H} W_h^2(\widehat{D}_h - D_h)^2\right] + \sum_{h=1}^{H}\sum_{i \neq h} W_h W_i \text{E}[(\widehat{D}_h - D_h)(\widehat{D}_i - D_i)] \\
&= \sum_h W_h^2 \text{var}[\widehat{D}_h] & (6.9) \\
&= \sum_h W_h^2 \text{E}_{c_h}[\text{var}(\widehat{D}_h \mid c_h)] & (6.10) \\
&= \sum_h W_h^2 \text{E}_{n_h}\left\{\frac{1}{a_h^2}[\text{var}(\overline{y}_h \mid n_h)]\right\}. & (6.11)
\end{aligned}
$$

If

$$
s_h^2 = \frac{1}{n_h - 1}\sum_{j=1}^{n_h}(y_{hj} - \overline{y}_h)^2,
$$

we have the usual unbiased estimate of $\text{var}[\overline{y}_h \mid n_h]$ and this leads to the unbiased estimate of $\text{var}[\widehat{D}]$, namely,

$$
\begin{aligned}
\widehat{\text{var}}[\widehat{D}] &= \sum_h W_h^2 \frac{s_h^2}{a_h^2 n_h}\left(1 - \frac{n_h}{N_h}\right) \\
&= \sum_h W_h^2 v_h, \quad \text{say.} & (6.12)
\end{aligned}
$$

It is interesting to note that the formulas (1.6) for nonadaptive stratified sampling are still unbiased for the adaptive allocation method.

Thompson and Seber (1996, p. 195) note that the above theory can be extended to the case when a_h also depends on c_h. We have that

$$
\text{E}[\widehat{D}_h \mid c_h] = \text{E}[\widehat{D}_h \mid n_h, a_h] = D_h,
$$

so that $\widehat{D}$ is still unbiased. Also $\text{var}[\widehat{D}]$ is still given by (6.10) and (6.11) if the expectation is with respect to both a_h and n_h. Then

$$
\text{E}[v_h] = \text{EE}[v_h \mid n_h, a_h]
$$

and $\widehat{\text{var}}[\widehat{D}]$ of (6.12) is still unbiased.

6.3 Some Adaptive Allocation Sampling Designs

We now consider some variations on our two-phase sampling theme. The appropriateness of a particular method depends very much on the population being sampled. The estimates obtained are generally biased, though the bias is usually small.

6.3.1 Francis's Design

Francis (1984), in his fisheries research, allocated his total fixed-sample size n to the strata in two phases, with the first-phase sample being $n_{.1}$ and the second-phase sample of size $n - n_{.1}$ being carried out in a sequential fashion. His design is based on a variance estimate of the total weight of fish (biomass) from the first phase for each stratum. When we estimate the stratum total biomass using a conventional estimator, the Francis's design is essentially equivalent to the following.

In allocating the second-phase sample we carry out the following steps for each unit. If an additional unit is added to stratum h, then, using the same estimate s_{h1}^2 from the first phase (defined in (6.1)), the reduction in the estimated variance of the conventional estimator is

$$G_h = N_h^2 (\frac{1}{n_{h1}} - \frac{1}{n_{h1} + 1}) s_{h1}^2 = \frac{N_h^2 s_{h1}^2}{n_{h1}(n_{h1} + 1)}.$$

This formula is now used to determine phase-2 allocations sequentially as follows. The first unit of the remaining unallocated units is allocated to the stratum for which G_h is the greatest. Suppose this is stratum j. Then G_j is recalculated as $N_j^2 s_{j1}^2 / (n_{j1} + 1)(n_{j1} + 2)$. The next unit is added to the stratum for which G_h is a maximum, and so on. Francis used the conventional stratified estimator which is biased. To control the bias, he suggested using $n_{.1} = (3/4)n$ for the phase-one sample.

6.3.2 Jolly-Hampton's Design

Jolly and Hampton (1990) proposed another adaptive allocation that can be formulated as a fixed sample-size design with n fixed again and $n_{.1}$ units in phase one. A first-phase sample of size n_{h1} is selected without replacement from each stratum h where n_{h1} is chosen such that $n_{h1} < n/H$. Variances of the strata are then estimated from this first-phase sample. The remaining $n - n_{.1}$ units are allocated as follows. The total sample size for the hth stratum is computed from

$$n_h = n_{h1} + (n - n_{.1}) \frac{N_h s_{h1}}{\sum_{h=1}^{H} N_h s_{h1}},$$

where s_{h1} is the standard deviation of the first-phase sample in the stratum h (see (6.1)). If the computed sample size in the hth stratum is larger than N_h, we select all the units in stratum h. They applied their method to an acoustic survey of South African anchovy.

6.3.3 Salehi-Smith's Design

Salehi and Smith (2005) introduced two-stage sequential sampling. In the special case that all the primary units are selected, the sampling design may be considered as an adaptive allocation design. In the first phase, a simple random sample is selected from each primary sample unit (stratum). To conduct the second phase, a condition C is defined for which the remaining sample size is allocated based on the value of the variable of interest. They used Murthy's estimator (Sect. 1.2.3), which is an unbiased estimator, for the population mean.

In the first phase a simple random sample of n_{h1} units is drawn without replacement from stratum h ($h = 1, \ldots, H$). If condition C is satisfied for at least one unit in the hth stratum in the first-phase sample, a predetermined number of additional units, say n_{h2}, are selected at random from the remaining units in stratum h. As a result $n = \sum_h n_{h1} + \sum_h n_{h2}$ is the total sample size, and is random. This method can be formulated as a variable sample-size design.

6.3.4 Brown et al.'s Method

Brown et al. (2008) introduced an adaptive allocation with a variable sample-size design that is more flexible than the Salehi-Smith design. The first phase is conducted as with the Salehi-Smith design, and a multiplier d is determined before sampling. In the second phase, if l_{h1} units from the first phase sample in stratum h satisfies the condition C, then additional $d \times l_{h1}$ units are sampled from the remaining units in stratum h. They used Murthy's estimator to estimate the population mean.

Moradi and Salehi (2010) modified Brown et al.'s method in which one selects one sample unit at least in the second phase regardless of the first-phase results. Murthy's estimator in Brown et al.'s sampling design is a weighted average with the weights calculated from the first-phase information only. They introduced a class of unbiased estimators for which the weights are calculated from both phases. They proved that the conventional estimator for stratified sampling is approximately unbiased. To estimate the variance of this estimator, they suggested two estimators. The first is the conventional stratified variance estimator, which is an under-estimate. The second is a bootstrap method similar to what Manly et al. (2002) introduced. A small study indicated that the bootstrap variance estimator is a slightly over-estimate.

6.3.5 Salehi et al.'s Method

Salehi et al. (2010) proposed a fixed sample-size version of Brown et al.'s method. The final sample size n is fixed, and a random sample of size n_{h1} ($h = 1, 2, \ldots, H$) is selected without replacement from each of the strata. Once again l_{h1} is the number of units in the first sample from stratum h that satisfy the condition C. Then d will be bounded and is given by

$$d = \frac{n - n_{.1}}{\sum_h l_{h1}},$$

where $n_{.1} = \sum_h n_{h1}$. We can select $d \times l_{h1}$ units from stratum h when $\sum_h l_{h1} > 0$, and then the final sample size would be equal to the predetermined sample size n. If $\sum_h l_{h1} = 0$, the multiplier d is undefined. To achieve a fixed sample size n, we allocate the remaining $n - \sum_h n_{h1}$ units equally to strata when $\sum_h l_{h1} = 0$. However, they noted that attaining the predetermined sample size n is not strictly true because of a rounding problem. The final sample size will be approximately equal to the predetermined sample size and may vary by a small amount depending on the effect of converting the real numbers to integers. They introduced a biased Horvitz-Thompson estimator and a biased sample-mean type of estimator for their method. They also recommended the latter for the Brown et al. method.

6.3.6 Complete Allocation Stratified Sampling

Salehi and Brown (2010) introduced a simplified adaptive allocation sampling design that targets the field effort and is logistically feasible. They called it complete allocation stratified sampling. It is an efficient and easily implemented adaptive sampling design.

Using stratification, let y_{hi} be the count of the species of interest in unit i from stratum h, let y_h be the stratum total count, and let τ be the total number of individuals in the population. Here the sample unit can be a plot, quadrat, or fisheries tow. In phase 1, a simple random sample of size n_h is taken without replacement from stratum h. The selected units are observed. If we observe any unit in stratum h that has a count of at least one, that is $y_h > 1$, all units in this stratum are selected. This selection of all units in the stratum is the second phase of sampling. For any strata in which all first-phase units have no individuals present, there is no second phase. As all observed units in these strata are zero, we can ignore them without losing any information. Let π_h be the probability that the entire stratum h is selected, that is, one of the nonempty units is selected. Suppose that m_h is the number of nonempty units in stratum h, then

$$\pi_h = 1 - \left[\binom{N_h - m_h}{n_h} \middle/ \binom{N_h}{n_h} \right].$$

Therefore the Horvitz-Thompson estimator of τ is

$$\widehat{\tau} = \sum_{h=1}^{\gamma} \frac{y_h^*}{\pi_h},$$

where y_h^* is the sum of the y_{hi} for the hth stratum, and γ is the number of strata for which at least one individual is observed in the first phase of sampling. Its variance is given by

$$\text{var}[\widehat{\tau}] = \sum_{h=1}^{H} \frac{(1 - \pi_h)y_h^{*2}}{\pi_h},$$

and an unbiased variance estimator is given by

$$\widehat{\text{var}}[\widehat{\tau}] = \sum_{h=1}^{\gamma} \frac{(1 - \pi_h)y_h^{*2}}{\pi_h^2}.$$

To evaluate the precision of complete allocation stratified sampling, Salehi and Brown (2010) used a modeled population of rockfish (*Sebates* species) in the Gulf of Alaska adopted from Su and Quinn II (2003). Results of the study with complete allocation stratified sampling showed high relative efficiency, especially if the survey is designed so that strata match the scale, and preferably shape, of aggregates in the population.

References

Brown J.A., M.M. Salehi, M. Moradi, G. Bell, and D. Smith. 2008. "Adaptive Two-Stage Sequential Sampling". *Population Ecology* 50:239–245.

Cochran, W.G. 1977. *Sampling Techniques*, 3rd edit. New York: Wiley.

Francis, R.I.C.C. 1984. "An Adaptive Strategy for Stratified Random Trawl Survey". *New Zealand Journal of Marine and Freshwater Research* 18:59–71.

Jolly, G.M., and I. Hampton. 1990. "A Stratified Random Transect Design for Acoustic Surveys of Fish Stocks". *Canadian Journal of Fisheries and Aquatic Science* 47:1282–1291.

Kremers, W.K. 1987. "Adaptive Sampling to Account for Unknown Variability Among Strata." Preprint No. 128. Institut für Mathematik, Universität Augsburg, Germany.

Manly, B.F.J., J.M. Akroyd, and K.A.R. Walshe. 2002. "Two-Phase Stratified Random Surveys on Multiple Populations at Multiple Locations". *New Zealand Journal of Marine and Freshwater Research* 36:581–591.

Moradi M., and M.M. Salehi. 2010. "An Adaptive Allocation Sampling Design for Which the Conventional Stratified Estimator is an Appropriate Estimator". *Journal of Statistical Planning and Inference* 140(4):1030–1037.

Su Z., and T.J. Quinn II. 2003. "Estimator Bias and Efficiency for Adaptive Cluster Sampling with Order Statistics and a Stopping Rule". *Environmental and Ecological Statistics* 10:17–41.

Salehi, M.M., and J.A. Brown. 2010. "Complete Allocation Sampling: An Efficient and Easily Implemented Adaptive Sampling Design". *Population Ecology* 52(3):451–456.

Salehi M.M., and D.R. Smith. 2005. "Two-Stage Sequential Sampling". *Journal of Agricultural, Biological, and Environmental Statistics* 10:84–103.

Salehi M.M., M. Moradi, J.A. Brown, and D.R. Smith. 2010. "Efficient Estimators for Adaptive Stratified Sequential Sampling". *Journal of Statistical Computation and Simulation* 80(10):1163–1179.

Thompson, S.K., F.L. Ramsey, and G.A.F. Seber. 1992. "An Adaptive Procedure for Sampling Animal Populations". *Biometrics* 48:1196–1199.

Thompson, S. K., and G.A.F. Seber. 1996. *Adaptive Sampling*. New York: Wiley.